MAKING CONNECTIONS WITH OTHERS:

A Handbook on Interpersonal Practice

Participant Manual

Debora Davidson, MS, OTR, BCP
Instructor
Program in Occupational Therapy
Washington University School of Medicine
St. Louis, Missouri

Suzanne M. Peloquin, PhD, OTR, FAOTA
Professor
Department of Occupational Therapy
School of Allied Health Sciences
University of Texas Medical Branch at Galveston
Galveston, Texas

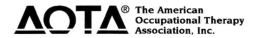
AOTA® The American Occupational Therapy Association, Inc.

Mission Statement

The mission of the American Occupational Therapy Association is to support a professional community for members, and to develop and preserve the viability and relevance of the profession. The organization serves the interest of its members, represents the profession to the public, and promotes access to occupational therapy services.

Vision Statement

AOTA leads occupational therapy as the preeminent profession recognized by all global communities of interest as having the scientific knowledge and expertise to promote and improve the health, productivity, and quality of life of individuals, communities, and society through the therapeutic application of occupation.

Disclaimers

"This publication is designed to provide accurate and authoritative information in regard to the subject matter covered. It is sold or distributed with the understanding that the publisher is not engaged in rendering legal, accounting, or other professional service. If legal advice or other expert assistance is required, the services of a competent professional person should be sought."

> —From the Declaration of Principles jointly adopted by the American Bar Association and a Committee of Publishers and Associations.

It is the objective of the American Occupational Therapy Association to be a forum for free expression and interchange of ideas. The opinions and positions expressed by the contributors to this work are their own and not necessarily those of either the editors or the American Occupational Therapy Association.

AOTA® Director of Nonperiodical Publications: Frances E. McCarrey
AOTA® Managing Editor of Nonperiodical Publications: Mary C. Fisk
Text design: World Composition Services, Inc.
Cover design: Irene Z Designs

Printed in the United States of America

ISBN 1-56900-100-6

Table of Contents

I. Introduction

Since we launched our course on interpersonal skills at the University of Texas Medical Branch at Galveston, we have shared its development with occupational therapists gathered at local and national conferences. At these we received many requests for more information about the objectives and resources that shaped the course. In response, we wrote an article that appeared in the March 1993 issue of the *American Journal of Occupational Therapy*. After reading the article, several educators pressed us for specifics about the activities that structure the course sessions. In response, we created a *Facilitator Manual* that allows individuals to replicate the course in clinical or academic settings. This *Participant Manual* is an attempt to respond to those who want to participate in this course in various settings and then to reproduce some of its activities.

The course works well in many settings. It has been offered both as an academic class and as a weekend workshop for practitioners. The 15 modules, each consisting of a reflection hour and a practice hour, may be offered sequentially or may stand alone. The modules may be structured as an intensive weekend workshop or as a series of continuing education opportunities for practitioners in clinical sites.

Rationale and Process: An Elaboration and Review

To review our overall aims in developing this course please refer to the article, "Interpersonal Skills for Practice: An Elective Course," which is reprinted in the Readings section. Other articles reprinted in that section should give insight into the thinking behind the evolution of the course. For example, "Communications Skills: Why Not Turn to a Training Model?" offers a rationale for designing a course that asks participants to reflect on practice and to be sensitive to the perspective of others. "Using the Arts to Enhance Confluent Learning" shares the reasoning behind the use of visual and literary arts in an interpersonal course. "Art: An Occupation with Promise for Developing Empathy" describes the characteristics of art that help develop an empathic disposition. "Sustaining the Art of Practice" recommends the use of fiction as a basis for discussion. "The Patient–Therapist Relationship in Occupational Therapy: Understanding Visions and Images" describes many nonfiction works used in this course and the rationale for their inclusion.

The use of self and the development of empathy—both aspects of the art of practice—are fundamental to the profession of occupational therapy as well as to other helping professions. The article "The Fullness of Empathy: Reflections and Illustrations" exemplifies the unique role of empathy in the practice of occupational therapy. Care delivery systems often press for practices that yield efficiency and productivity rather than the interpersonal interactions that are perceived by patients as caring. In "The Depersonalization of Patients: A Profile Gleaned from Narratives" are numerous descriptions of the helper behaviors that are problematic in this way; a companion article, "The Patient–Therapist Relationship: Beliefs That Shape Care," discusses the pressures that caregivers encounter and the societal beliefs that shape these pressures. "Now That We Have Managed Care, Shall We Inspire It?" offers hope and direction to those who practice within systems that disregard the ethos of caring.

Organization and Use of the Facilitator and Participant Manuals

We created two manuals for this course. The Facilitator Manual contains surprise exercises, suggested responses to questions, excerpts from most readings, the hidden agendas within role plays, and a final evaluation. The Participant Manual is an abbreviated version of the Facilitator Manual. Using this manual, participants can ready themselves for each session by skimming the basic themes and questions that structure each session and by reading recommended articles.

Separate introductions precede both the reflection and practice hours in each manual. Each introduction contains the guidelines and principles that structure both components of the course.

Our goal in making this course available is to share a process that has been effective for us and has been well received by various audiences. We hope that each user of this manual will take some of what we offer, use it, reflect on it, but, in the end, create his or her own personalized version. To this end, we warmly invite your comments and suggestions.

II. Guidelines for the Reflection Hour

This hour aims to evoke reflection. It should be shaped by the thoughts and feelings of the participants. The facilitator's role is to introduce experiences that will evoke discourse, enhance personal and interpersonal understanding, and shape an empathic disposition.

The Participant Manual has been designed so as to offer a preview of the major themes of each session without revealing the surprise element of the exercises or readings. The Participant Manual has abbreviated excerpts from readings contained in the Facilitator Manual; it directs participants to the references from which facilitators will read. The format of the Participant Manual also gives learners enough direction to replicate the sessions in their practice if they wish to do so later.

Resources for the reflection hours can be found through local libraries or through interlibrary loan from a university library. Participants are encouraged to supplement the readings in this manual with others from the Readings section, which are briefly annotated below:

1. The Depersonalization of Patients: A Profile Gleaned from Narratives
   - Many stories that patients have told about difficult experiences with caregivers
   - A sampling of stories describing what patients want instead

2. The Fullness of Empathy: Reflections and Illustrations
   Several examples of caring and empathic behaviors in occupational therapy from the life of Ora Ruggles, a reconstruction aide

3. The Patient–Therapist Relationship: Understanding visions and Images
   Examples of phenomenological stories about patients who have had positive experience with their occupational therapists as technicians, parents, or covenanted friends

4. Sustaining the Art of Practice in Occupational Therapy
   - Several examples from the fictional literature of therapists' positive and negative exchanges with patients
   - Several examples of the positive effect of occupation used therapeutically

III. Guidelines for Participation in Role Playing

This part of the course is based on a behavioral-learning model and is designed to help the participants become increasingly competent and comfortable. Each participant begins with unique inherent abilities and experiences, and groups of participants may possess a wide range of competencies. The main goal is for each individual to achieve basic concepts and beginning-to-intermediate skills in therapeutic relating.

All participants are expected to engage in a variety of role-play exercises and to play a variety of parts. Participants may be asked to take turns around the circle or to volunteer on a regular basis.

Even the most poised individuals usually approach role playing with some trepidation. Although such anxiety is uncomfortable, it is healthy and normal and will likely decrease with experience. The teacher–facilitator will use a variety of techniques to develop participants' increasing comfort with the process. Participants can help speed this process by

- acknowledging these emotions and interacting with one another in a mutually supportive manner

- recognizing that role playing has been thoroughly researched and found to be an effective method for developing social skills

- desensitizing themselves to performance anxiety by speaking during the discussion portions of the sessions and participating in the "warm-up" phases of the course

- focusing attention on classmates' role-play performance and offering assistance as a coach

- trying a variety of roles, including those of clients or colleagues, as well as therapists

- keeping things in perspective and enjoying the opportunity to make mistakes without negative consequences and

- remembering that there are many effective ways to approach any of the situations presented.

Participants should be challenged to explore and learn through trial-and-error in a safe environment that does not distress participants to or make them feel incompetent. Role plays are designed to elicit risk taking, problem solving, and discussion.

In contrast to the real world, the therapist in role play is never alone. All those present are potential coaches, who may offer or be asked for ideas at any time. The therapist should feel free to stop the action or "rewind" and repeat it as needed. The instructor may also take this liberty if the role play needs an adjustment.

To increase the realism of the role plays, the perspectives of the clients and colleagues in the role plays are found only in the Facilitators Manual. The facilitator will share these descriptions with the role players before starting each scenario. It is important to have fun with the roles and to act emotionally or irrationally, if that is what the role calls for. Clients should strive to challenge the therapist, but only to the point that it feels natural. Effective communication usually produces an urge to cooperate (or at least to calm down and try to communicate). When that urge is elicited, it is best to act on it. Otherwise, it is best to keep on challenging the therapist.

IV. The Course

Session 1: Becoming Personal and Professional

Reflection Hour

This session differs from the other reflection hours because it aims both to evoke reflection and to introduce the course. The pace of this hour will be brisker than in subsequent reflection hours.

1. Review the course syllabus. The course explores three major concepts from the occupational therapy literature: art of practice, use of self, and empathy.

2. Discuss the concepts fundamental to any practice among persons.

    Adler, A. (1931). *What life should mean to me* (p. 36). Boston: Little, Brown.

    Mosey, A. C. (1981). The art of practice. *Occupational therapy: Configuration of a profession* (p. 22). New York: Raven Press.

    Tiffany, F. G. (1988). The therapeutic use of self. Hopkins, H.L. & Smith, H. D. (Eds.), *Willard and Spackman's occupational therapy* (7th ed., p. 316). Philadelphia: Lippincott.

3. Tubesing's schema for developing empathy nicely illustrates the approach or methodology of the course. Discuss Tubesing's schema.

    See Tubesing, D. A., & Tubesing, N. L. (1973). *Tune-in—Empathy training workshop.* Duluth, MN: Listening Group.

    Connect the schema to the process of this course:

    The *Reflection Hour* of this course emphasizes tuning in to and expressing the self.

    The *Practice Hour* of this course emphasizes tuning in to and responding to others.

4. Discuss the limitations of approaches that teach communication as technique rather than as an attitude and presence. See Plum, A. (1981). Communication as skill: A critique and alternative. *Humanistic Psychology, 21*, 3–19.

    This course aims to foster the attitude and presence that are fundamental to skilled interactions. Refer to S. M. Peloquin's "Communication skills: Why not turn to a skills training model?," *American Journal of Occupational Therapy* in the Readings Section.

5. Face the awkwardness involved in a course that puts oneself on display. This course may create some awkward moments as participants share reflections and practice ways of interacting with others. The following exercise aims to start the process in a spirit of mutual helpfulness and willingness to grow.

    Complete the exercise and discuss
    • What are the positive and negative functions of a mask?

6. Explore the accusation that helpers wear a professional mask.

    Discuss how being both personal and professional in practice means to have integrity or to be real. Then discuss the underlying request that helpers *try* to understand others or be empathic, and try to be real and open or assertive with them. Read about the process of understanding. See Sarason, S. (1985). *Caring and compassion in clinical practice*. San Francisco: Jossey-Bass.

    This course will ask participants to move freely between being empathic and being assertive in practice.

Options and Alternatives

There is a challenge in being personal and real. Engage in open discussion about the topic. Discuss excerpts from any of the following:

Consider

Adler, R., & Towne, N. (1992). "Please hear what I'm not saying" *Looking out/looking in*. New York: Holt, Rhinehart, and Winston. Discuss the "wearing of a mask" in this context.

Beisser, A. (1989). [title of chapter]. *Flying without wings: Personal reflections on becoming disabled* (p. 35). New York: Doubleday. Arnold Beisser discusses hospital caretakers who leave patients unattended to take their coffee breaks.

Prather, H. (1972). *I touch the earth, the earth touches me*. New York: Doubleday.

Slaby, A. A., & Glickman, A. S. (1986). Adaptation of physicians to managing life-threatening illness. *Integrative Psychiatry, 4*, 162–165. Andrew Slaby and Arvin Glickman discuss stainless-steel hearts in practice.

Recommendation

Read "Interpersonal Skills for Practice: An Elective Course" from the Readings section.

Session 1: **Becoming Personal and Professional**

Practice Hour

1. Introduction: Discuss the benefits of having a variety of communication styles from which to choose when approaching challenging situations with clients and colleagues.

2. Complete the Communication Styles Analysis Worksheet with the group.

3. Review the Log Assignments that are numbered to correspond with the session topics.

4. Review the Assertiveness Self-Rating Inventory. Complete this worksheet before the next session.

5. Review the Challenging Interpersonal Interactions Journal. This will be used for some log assignments and may be used throughout the course as a personal log of your development.

Figure 2. Communication Styles Analysis Worksheet

	AGGRESSIVE	passive	passive-AGGRESSIVE	Assertive
Verbal				
Tone				
Movements				
Thoughts				
Feelings				
Benefits				
Costs				

Log Assignments

Week 1

Complete the Assertiveness Self-Rating Inventory. Keep a weeklong journal in which you chart your responses to challenging interpersonal situations, using the Challenging Interpersonal Interactions Journal form. Record 3 to 5 interactions.

Week 2

Compose a dialogue of a challenging situation involving yourself and one or two other characters. The situation may be reality-based (even borrowed from last week's journal) or fictional. It may involve efforts to coerce, ridicule, or otherwise manipulate you. Write the dialogue so that your character responds assertively.

Week 3

Use an active listening style several times this week in daily interactions, and write a paragraph describing the interaction, outcome, and your feelings about the experience.

Week 4

Find magazine photos of at least 10 people and write captions describing the emotions you think the people are expressing. Seek full-body pictures.

Week 5

Use an active listening style with someone who is expressing anger, frustration, fatigue, or other emotions of distress. Write a paragraph describing the interaction, its outcome, and your reactions.

Week 6

Recall a time when you have had to say no, and describe the interaction. If you feel that your communication style could have been improved, rewrite the story to reflect an ideal outcome.

Week 7

Describe your worst fear about interviewing. Do you worry about clients' tearfulness, anger, silence, flirtation, body odor, and so forth? Imagine the worst possible scenario involving this fear. Write a paragraph or dialogue in which you deal effectively with such a situation.

Week 8

As an occupational therapist, what information would you find it difficult to share with a client or the client's family? What are your fears about such an interaction? How would you prepare yourself and set up the interaction to go as successfully as possible?

Week 9

Imagine a treatment team consisting of a health administrator, a physician, a psychologist/ researcher, a speech pathologist, a nurse, a social worker, a personal care aide, a spouse, a physical therapist, and an occupational therapist. The client is a 25-year-old man who has moved into a residential rehabilitation facility after having incurred a severe brain injury from an auto accident. The client is in a wheelchair and is currently confused and combative. List what you think each team member's main concerns and goals for the client might be. Include the client as a team member.

Week 10

Recall a time when you were in conflict with a peer or authority figure. Identify the overt and hidden agendas of the parties involved. How could respect for the other person's needs have been conveyed?

Week 11

Respond to criticism using negative inquiry and report on the interaction. Include the verbal and behavioral exchange and your feelings about it.

Week 12

Provide corrective feedback to someone in an assertive, positive manner. (This may be spontaneous or in a role play.) Afterward, ask the other person for feedback regarding your style. (For example, were you clear, specific, positive, and helpful?) Report on the interaction and the emotional reactions of you and the other person.

Week 13

Describe a time when you or your work were criticized by a peer or by a person in authority. What was—or was not—helpful? Would you like to rewrite your part? If so, how?

Week 14

Write a paragraph about your reaction to this course as a whole. Was it what you hoped? How, or how not? Do you think that your practice as an occupational therapist will be influenced by what you have experienced in the classes? If so, how?

Week 15

Prepare for an essay.

Assertiveness Self-Rating Inventory

U = Usually difficult S = Sometimes difficult N = Rarely difficult **BEHAVIORS**	**PERSONS**	**Authority figures:** supervisor, teacher, administrator, physician	**Colleagues/peers**	**Subordinates:** supervisees, students	**Business contacts:** salespersons, office workers	**Patients/clients:** elderly	**Patients/clients:** adults
Express positive feelings, give compliments							
Receive compliments							
Make requests, e.g., ask for favors, help, etc.							
Express liking, affection							
Initiate and maintain conversation							
Compliment yourself							
Stand up for your rights							
Refuse requests							
Express personal opinions including disagreement							
Express negative feelings							
Express justified annoyance and displeasure							
Express justified anger							

Challenging Interpersonal Interactions Journal

Directions

Keeping a journal is a time-honored way of increasing one's awareness of feelings and thoughts, and can help in the quest to change behavioral patterns. As soon as possible after their occurrence, write down examples of interactions that you have found difficult or stressful, and analyze your feelings and the pieces of the exchange that did, or did not, seem successful. This will help you develop self-awareness, encourage you in trying new skills, and allow you to celebrate your successes. You may want to make extra copies of the blank form for future use.

Challenging Interpersonal Interactions Journal

Date: _____

The setting: _____

The situation: _____

_____

_____

_____

I said . . . because . . . : _____

_____

My physical reactions were: _____

My observable behaviors were: _____

_____

My emotions were: _____

The other person was probably feeling . . . , because . . . : _____

_____

Ideally, my response to this situation would be to: _____

_____

_____

Adapted with permission from Bloom, L. Z. et al. (1975). *The new assertive woman.* New York: Delacorte Press.

Challenging Interpersonal Interactions Journal

Date: *December 24, 1996*

The setting: *A crowded restaurant*

The situation: *It took 45 minutes to be served a salad, which turned out to have the wrong dressing and spoiled lettuce in it. The waiter was rude and made himself unavailable.*

I said . . . because . . . : *Nothing, because I didn't want to make a scene.*

My physical reactions were: *Upset stomach, cheeks felt hot*

My observable behaviors were: *Sighing, frowning, mumbling curses; left small tip*

My emotions were: *Anger, frustration, intimidation*

The other person was probably feeling . . . , because . . . : *Apathetic. Unaware of my anger, because I did not say anything.*

Ideally, my response to this situation would be to: *Walk over to the manager and ask for better service before I became so angry and was late for work, or go to a less crowded place at the outset.*

Adapted with permission from Bloom, L. Z. et al. (1975). *The new assertive woman.* New York: Delacorte Press.

Session 2: The Therapeutic Use of Self

Reflection Hour

1. Consider the concept of the continuum of conscious/therapeutic use of self. See Hopkins, H. L. & Smith, H. D. (Eds.). (1988). *Willard and Spackman's occupational therapy*. Philadelphia: Lippincott.

2. Discuss the concept of art as "making something" of a world-experience, a process that satisfies rules of harmony and balance while it illuminates some aspect of reality. Understand that a fictional story may be based on some experience that is transformed into a work of art.

   Consider the story "Brute" from Richard Selzer's fictional work. See Selzer, R. (1982). *Letters to a young doctor*. New York: Simon & Schuster, pp. 59–63. This powerful story takes about 8 minutes to read. Note closely the doctor's thoughts, feelings, and actions.

   Discuss from among the following questions:

   • How would you characterize the problem?

   • What factors led up to the problem (That is, actions, attitudes, and feelings)?

   • Who is the "brute" in this story?

   • What kinds of actions might have changed the course of this encounter or defused the situation?

   • What possible real life incidents might have inspired the writing of this story?

   Consider another nonfictional account. See Holderly, R. & McNulty, E. (1982). *Treating and caring: A human approach to patient care* (pp. 91–92). Reston, VA: Reston Publishing. This story closely parallels the artistic rendition in "Brute."

   The conscious use of self, as reflected in Selzer's work, consists of one's awareness of situations that might cause problems. Briefly discuss the following:

   • What incidents or attitudes might be problematic for you?

   • What does your "brute" look like?

   Most reflection hours and the log experiences will invite participants to make some personal disclosure, especially as the course progresses.

3. Consider James Thurber's fable "The Hen Who Wouldn't Fly." See Thurber, J. (1940). *Fables for our times*. New York: Harper Brothers. Connect the fable's moral with the "use of self."

Recommendation

Read "Communication skills: Why not turn to a training model" from the Readings section.

Session 2: **The Therapeutic Use of Self**

Practice Hour

1. Briefly review the benefits of getting to know one's own style ("tuning into ourselves") in order to reach effectiveness in communicating with others.

2. Color code your responses on the Communication Style Self-Rating Inventory.

3. Describe how patterns of relative comfort and skill emerge and share with the group a pattern that you see in your profile. For example, a band of red down Column A indicates generalized difficulty in interacting with people in positions of authority. This may cause avoidance or friction when dealing with supervisors. A stripe of red and yellow across the "refuse requests" row reflects a problem that may cause the respondent to become swamped with obligations.

4. Review the Rights and Responsibilities of Assertive Persons, next page.

5. Participate in a brief role play related to setting limits. Then give yourself a pat on the back for surviving your first role play!

Rights and Responsibilities of Assertive Persons

All persons' ideas and feelings deserve equal respect.

Everyone's needs are equally important.

Each of us chooses when he or she wishes to be responsible for supplying solutions to others' problems.

All persons have the right to change their minds.

All persons have the right to make mistakes. Each of us is responsible for his or her actions but need not feel devastated by errors.

It is acceptable not to know everything and to admit ignorance.

Each of us chooses with whom to agree and whom to like.

It is acceptable not to be liked or agreed with by everyone.

All persons have the right to make illogical decisions regarding personal matters.

It is not always necessary to explain or justify our actions to others.

Each of us has the right and responsibility to judge the appropriateness of our emotions, thinking, and behavior and to make changes in ourselves as needed.

It is acceptable to refuse the goodwill of others.

Rights	Responsibilities
To speak up	To listen
To take	To give
To have problems	To find solutions
To be comforted	To comfort others
To work	To do one's best
To make mistakes	To correct mistakes
To criticize	To praise
To be rewarded	To reward others
To be independent	To be depended on
To cry	To dry tears
To be loved	To love others

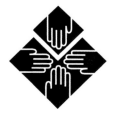

Session 3: **Active Listening**

Reflection Hour

1. Consider the questions that the facilitator will ask relative to personal preferences. Answer the first question. Review Adler's definition of empathy from Session 1: *Empathy is the common sense that we have of one another.* See Adler, A. (1931). *What life should mean to you.* Boston: Little, Brown. Review the notion that empathy builds on likeness and universality of experience and consider whether the answers to the first question supported that view.

    Answer the second question. Comment on Adler's definition and try to make a connection with the title of this session, "Active Listening." Active listening to individual differences is also essential for true understanding.

2. Consider James Thurber's fable "The Scotty Who Knew Too Much." See Thurber, J. (1940). *Fables for our times.* New York: Harper Brothers (33–34). Discuss the moral of the story, "It is better to ask some of the questions than to know all of the answers" (p. 30) within the context of active listening.

3. Consider what Hodgins said about real listening. See Hodgins, E. (1964). Whatever became of the healing art? *Annals of the New York Academy of Sciences,* 164, 838–840.

4. Look at a reproduction of the abstract painting *Burned face* by Dutch artist Karl Appel. See Janson, H. W. (1986). History of art (Rev. ed.). Englewood, NJ: Prentice-Hall (p. 695). Simultaneously consider an excerpt from Suzanne Peloquin's dissertation. See Peloquin, S. M. (1991). *Art in practice: When art becomes caring* (pp. 278–285). Galveston: University of Texas Medical Branch, Moody Medical Library. The text aims to lead to an empathic connection with one another and to illustrate the foundation of active listening—the willingness to understand.

    Discuss the following:

    • Have you ever spent this long a time thinking about a painting?

    • What was the experience like?

    • Did you hear or see anything that you would have missed if you had just glanced at the work on a museum wall?

    • How is this exercise like active listening?

    • What are the benefits and risks of active listening?

    • What are the obstacles to active listening in practice?

5. Discuss the assigned reading "Communication Skills: Why Not Turn to a Training Model?" from the Readings section.

Options and Alternatives

Find the book *Healing and the Mind.* See Moyers, B. (1993). *Healing and the Mind.* New York: Doubleday. Look at the picture of Alfredo Casteneda's *Consideration* on p. 346. Select any popular song that deals with listening or not listening. Look at the reproduction of the painting while listening to the song.

Recommendation

Read "The Patient–Therapist Relationship: Understanding Visions and Images" from the Readings section.

Session 3: **Active Listening**

Practice Hour

This session marks the beginning of structured role playing. The scenarios increase in complexity and challenge from session to session and reflect the general topic of each section. They are drawn from clinical experience in a variety of settings and may be supplemented with, or replaced by, experiences that the participants wish to share.

1. The facilitator will read aloud the background information from a scenario and will ask for volunteers to play the student/therapist and the other character (initially this will be a client; later it will be a colleague or supervisor). The student/therapist will read aloud the information provided while the person playing the other character will read that part silently. The teacher may want to step out of the room to coach the "client" on how to play the role to its best advantage. During the role play, the "therapist" may stop the action at any time to solicit advice from those fellow participants who are designated as coaches. The teacher may also choose to stop the action in order to shape it but should try to let the group work things out as much as possible.

2. Review the Active Listening instructions that follow.

3. Begin role playing.

Active Listening

Active listening is a communication technique that

- Demonstrates respect for and value of others
- Facilitates accurate information-gathering
- Contributes to the therapeutic process

THE ACTIVE LISTENER WILL FOCUS COMPLETE ATTENTION ON THE SPEAKER

Communicate interest with

- Eye contact
- Posture
- Facial expression
- Movement
- Vocal expressions

Paraphrase what was said, including affect and content

- "You feel . . . because . . . "
- "It seems to you that . . . "
- "As I hear it, you feel . . . because . . . "
- "Perhaps you're feeling . . . "
- "It sounds like you're feeling . . . "
- "That sounds really . . . How do you feel about it?"

Seek confirmation or clarification

- "Does that fit?"
- "Is that an accurate guess?"
- "Does that describe you?"

Offer empathy and support

- "I know this is difficult."
- "That sounds so stressful."
- "I want to help you feel better."
- "That's incredible!"
- "I'm concerned about you."

Explore events and feelings further

- "What else is going on?"
- "What are your feelings when that occurs?"
- "Tell me what else you remember."
- "Try to recall what you felt at the moment."

Facilitate the other's problem solving

- "How can I be of help?"

- "What are some of your options at this time?"

- "What have you tried?"

- "What are your thoughts at this point?"

Active listening does **not** include

- Giving Advice
  "Why don't you . . . ?", "Have you . . . ?"

- Correcting
  "I'm sure he didn't mean . . . "

- Invalidating
  "Don't worry . . . " or "You can handle it!"

Session 3: **Active Listening**

Role Play

Scenario A: Adolescent Anger

Background: The client is a 15-year-old who was admitted to an inpatient mental health unit the previous day with a history of truancy, running away from home, alcohol abuse, and suicidal ideation. This hospitalization was initiated when the client's mother discovered that the teenager had been drinking on a daily basis and was romantically involved with a 40-year-old neighbor. This is your first meeting.

Therapist: You want to begin establishing rapport while learning about your client's thoughts and feelings related to being hospitalized and the problems at home. You see a sullen-looking teenager wearing torn jeans, a "Megadeth" T-shirt, multiple earrings, and a tattoo. Despite the tough exterior, there is an air of lonely isolation about this child.

Session 3: **Active Listening**

Role Play

Scenario B: The Reluctant Chef

Background: The 68-year-old patient is in rehabilitation for upper extremity weakness and low endurance after a cervical spinal laminectomy. The patient is a retired vice-president of a large metropolitan bank and has been active in a variety of community and cultural activities. The patient is married and has children and grandchildren living in the same city. Prior to today, the patient has been motivated and good humored in occupational therapy. According to the rehabilitation unit's protocol, today the patient must complete the cold food preparation evaluation, which entails making and serving a tuna salad sandwich. The rehabilitation team is optimistic about a full recovery.

Therapist: You want to understand your patient's concerns and to ascertain what is bothering the patient. You would like to proceed with the cooking evaluation, but you do not want to sacrifice your rapport with the patient.

Session 3: **Active Listening**

Role Play

Scenario C: New World I

Background: A 22-year-old man has been home for 1 month following rehabilitation for a spinal cord injury incurred in an auto accident caused by his driving while intoxicated. He is paraplegic and has no motor or sensory functioning below T-7. The outpatient occupational therapist is meeting with the patient's parent, who has been looking increasingly distressed since the patient's discharge from the inpatient program. The patient has missed several sessions this week, has been irritable and unmotivated in occupational therapy, and has deteriorated in his grooming.

Therapist: You can see that things are not going well at home. You are meeting with the patient to try to find out what the problems are and to provide an opportunity to explore his feelings. Begin by saying something like, "Let's take a moment to talk about how things are going at home."

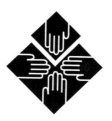

Session 4: **Nonverbal Communication**

Reflection Hour

1. Look at two or three of Gary Larson's cartoons that relate to eye contact or touch. Larson, G. (1991). *Unnatural selections.* Kansas City: Universal Press. or *The far side gallery* see Larson G. (1986, 1988). Kansas City: Andrews and McMeel.

2. Discuss the distinctions between instrumental touch and expressive touch:

    • When do occupational therapists use touch instrumentally?

    • When might it be appropriate to use touch expressively? What body parts are *safe* to touch?

    • What situations and kinds of touch are either inappropriate or pose a high risk of misunderstanding?

3. Consider excerpts (in particular, pp. 40–41 and pp. 90–96) from a book by Victor Small. The story is a humorous illustration of a young caregiver's having witnessed the almost magical use of touch by an aide and then trying to work the magic himself. The setting is a mental health facility in the early part of this century: See Small, V. (1935). *I knew 3,000 lunatics.* New York: Ferris Printing. The recommended excerpts should take about 5 to 7 minutes to read.

    • What went wrong in this encounter?

    • Consider this comment from Sir Dominic Corrigan: "The trouble with doctors is not that they don't know enough, but that they don't see enough." What signs did the young doctor fail to see or hear? See Taylor, R. B. (1972). The practical art of medicine. New York: Harper & Row.

    • Consider this question: On a scale of 1 to 10, how comfortable are you with touching others? Consider the same question about your comfort level with being touched. Discuss the implications of individual comfort levels relative to the needs of patients.

4. Discuss "The Patient-Therapist Relationship: Understanding Visions and Images" from the Readings section

Options and Alternatives

Consider the short story "Pinch." The story is about instrumental touch during a mammogram. Discuss the absence of human connection in this encounter. Discuss the instances of touch and the messages that were, or were not, communicated through these. See Oates, J. C. (1988). *The assignation.* New York: Ecco Press, pp. 65–67.

Use a videotape of any television sitcom. Consider the instances in which touch was instrumental or expressive. Discuss whether there were instances in which instrumental and expressive touch merged.

Recommendation

Read "Sustaining the Art of Practice" from the Readings section.

Session 4: **Nonverbal Communication**

Practice Hour

1. Brainstorm the variety of ways that nonverbal communication takes place between therapists and clients.

2. Discuss nonverbal communication as a powerful therapeutic tool that may be used to receive, send, and understand information. Briefly discuss how nonverbal communication is a central part of active listening.

3. Some therapeutic techniques like those below involve nonverbal communication:

   • Try subtly mirroring some of your client's movements and facial expressions when encouraging self-disclosure and trust. Use head nodding.

   • Relax your posture and slow your breathing rate when trying to calm an agitated client. Try matching the breathing rate of a client whose activity is slowed because of depression or sadness. Use a calm, lowered voice in both instances.

   • Observe for mismatched verbal or nonverbal communications (for example, "I'm not upset!" said with clenched fists; or "I'm pleased to meet you," said with eyes averted and a slightly wrinkled nose.) A mismatch may reflect unconscious conflict or intentional reticence. The therapist may choose simply to note the mismatch, follow up with indirect probing, or to directly address the process (for example, by stating, "You are saying that you are not upset, but you are clenching your fists and looking angry.")

4. Go on to role plays. Strive to use nonverbal as well as verbal communication skills.

Session 4: **Nonverbal Communication**

Role Play

Scenario A: Confused Cookie

Background: The client is a 35-year-old who is seeking help for work-related carpal tunnel syndrome. After surgery, 4 weeks ago, the patient was given a splint designed to facilitate healing, along with specific instructions about limitations on activity and ways to exercise properly. The patient missed 3 of the last 4 occupational therapy sessions, and has made little improvement.

Therapist: You are confused by this patient's lack of progress and cooperation, despite the professed desire to return to work. You want to facilitate a positive working relationship while sorting out the events, feelings, and behaviors that have resulted the lack of improvement. (*Clinical hint*: Bowling is *not* a recommended activity for persons recovering from carpal tunnel surgery!)

Session 4: **Nonverbal Communication**

Role Play

Scenario B: New World II

Background: A 22-year-old man has been home for 1 month following rehabilitation for a spinal cord injury received in an accident caused by his driving while intoxicated. He is paraplegic and has no motor or sensory functioning below T-7. The outpatient occupational therapist is meeting with the patient and his parent, who has been looking increasingly distressed since the patient's discharge from the inpatient program. The patient has missed several sessions this week, has been irritable and unmotivated in occupational therapy, and has deteriorated in his grooming. You are meeting with the client and his parent.

Therapist: You can see that things are not going well at home and you have been unable to get much information from your patient. You are meeting with the patient and his parent to try to find out what the problems are and to provide an opportunity for them to explore their feelings and get some support. Begin by saying something like, "Let's take a moment to talk about how things are going at home."

Session 4: **Nonverbal Communication**

Role Play

Scenario C: Elementary Upset

Background: The client is a fifth-grade teacher. Recently, Joe, a student with severe cerebral palsy and an IQ of 120, was assigned to this classroom as part of a district-wide movement to include the disabled in regular classrooms. The school occupational therapist has been asked to consult with Joe's teacher regarding the student's special needs. The student will have a full-time aide who can assist with his physical care.

Therapist: The district's goal of integrating disabled students into regular classrooms is set and not debatable. Listen to this teacher's feelings, and work to uncover what lies beneath the surface emotions. Strive to create a supportive relationship while not compromising the district's plans. (*Note*: Solving the problem of the logistics of Joe's school performance is not needed at this point.)

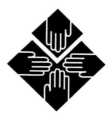

Session 5: **The Power of Feelings**

Reflection Hour

1. Discuss individual definitions of the word *feeling*.

2. Discuss the feelings that caregivers can anticipate having in practice.

3. Consider the short story "Pinch," which is about a woman's experience with caregivers who examine her breasts. See Oates, J. C. (1988). The assignation. New York: Ecco Press. Discuss from among the following questions:

   • What feelings do you think that the caregivers might have had?

   • Do the caregivers express their feelings? How, or how not?

   • Does the woman express her feelings during this exchange? How, or how not?

   • What meanings can you assign to the story's title, beyond the obvious pinch of the machine?

   • What kinds of feelings, beyond those already discussed, do you expect your patients or clients to have during your treatments? What feelings do you expect to have?

4. Discuss the consequences of a caregiver's expression of feelings, using the above story as a springboard.

   • What feelings do you anticipate that you will *want* to express to your patients/clients?

   • Are there feelings that you will want to "pinch"?

5. Discuss "Sustaining the Art of Practice" from the Readings section.

Options and Alternatives

Consider the moving segments (pp. 8–9 and pp. 18–19) from *Patient interviewing*. See Reiser, D., & Schroder, A. K. (1975). *Patient interviewing: The human dimension*. San Francisco: Institute for the Study of Humanistic Medicine. The scenario portrays the relationship between a medical student and a patient and his feelings upon learning of her death. Discuss questions from No. 3 above using this narrative as a springboard.

Recommendation

Read "The Depersonalization of Patients: A Profile Gleaned from Narratives" from the Readings section.

Session 5: **The Power of Feelings**

Practice Hour

The following role plays provide practice in responding to anger directed at the therapist, to anxiety, and to suicidal thoughts. Briefly review the key issues involved in screening for suicidal risk (for example, mood, vegetative symptoms, frequency of suicidal thoughts, and lethality of plan). Remember that you will be functioning as a member of a health care team.

Session 5: **The Power of Feelings**

Role Play

Scenario A: Adolescent Anger

Background: A 16-year-old who has been diagnosed with conduct disorder and depression is in residential care. Therapeutic rapport appeared to be positive until the last three sessions. During these, the client was verbally provocative (mumbling curse words when limits were set, arguing with therapist's directives, repeatedly hinting at plans to run away to the city to join a gang). The client also refused to participate in group activities. The therapist reported this behavior at a team meeting, as did other team members, and the team decided to revoke the client's weekend pass to visit his aunt.

Therapist: You notice that your client looks angry and withdrawn. You want to help him express his feelings, learn how to handle conflict effectively, and start to accept responsibility for his feelings and behavior. (Remember that you are a member of this patient's treatment team and not the sole decision-maker.)

Session 5: **The Power of Feelings**

Role Play

Scenario B: Anxious Elder

Background: The patient is a frail 88-year-old who is in inpatient rehabilitation after breaking a hip. The patient very much wants to return home but may need to enter a skilled care facility if he (or she) does not meet the goals of daily living activities within the next 2 weeks. The patient resists to trying any movements that require weight-bearing on the right leg, or weight shifting, and therefore has not yet been able to work on using the toilet, putting on pants or socks, or bathing. The patient has concerned family members but wants to continue living alone.

Therapist: You think that this patient has the physical and cognitive skills to regain functional independence. However, the patient's anxiety and resistance to therapy prevent working toward the agreed-upon goals of independent dressing, use of the toilet, and bathing. Your goal is to understand and, if possible, gain the patient's trust and cooperation. At this time, you approach the patient to transfer him (or her) to the wheelchair.

Session 5: **The Power of Feelings**

Role Play

Scenario C: Suicidal Behavior

Background: The patient is a 40-year-old who has been hospitalized repeatedly for major depression and attempts at suicide. Married and with three young children, the patient has a doctoral degree in computer science and works for an international corporation. The patient is in a projective activity group with four other patients and a therapist. The patient's drawing was done in black and red, featuring themes of death (crosses, open graves, and dead flowers). The patient refuses to describe the drawing to the group.

Therapist: You invite the patient to a separate area to talk. You want to assess the risk of suicide. Ask about thoughts, feelings, cognitive functioning (memory and concentration), and physical functioning (for example, eating, sleeping, and energy level). Gently probe for any possible precipitating life events. Explain your plan of intervention to the patient (for example, referral to the primary physician for full evaluation and notifying the head nurse for safety precautions on the unit). Express feelings of caring and hope for this patient and praise the patient for sharing these difficult feelings.

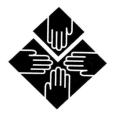

Session 6: **Tough Love**

Reflection Hour

1. Consider the cartoon by A. Zilinskas entitled "Relationships" (*New York Times*, Sunday, April 8, 1990). Look carefully at the picture and discuss what Zilinskas is saying about relationships. Look at the body language of the individuals. See Zilinskas, A. (1990, April 8). "Relationships." *The New York Times*.

   Discuss the phrase *tough love*.

   • What might tough love look like clinically?

   • What kinds of situations will warrant your tough love?

2. Consider two excerpts (see p. 7 and pp. 42–43) from a book by Barbara Benzinger. Discuss the interaction between the nurse and Benzinger in which the nurse sets limits in a rude way (pp. 34–35). See Benzinger, B. F. (1969). *The prison of my mind.* New York: Walker.

   Then consider the interaction between the patient and the occupational therapist in which the therapist allows Benzinger to keep a pair of scissors in her room as long as she follows certain guidelines. Make comparisons between the two caregivers in order to get a better sense of how limits can be set without damaging the patient.

3. Consider an excerpt (pp. 33–35) from Act 1 of a play by B. Clark. Reflect about the conversation between the paralyzed patient, Ken, and the social worker, Mrs. Boyle. The social worker talks to Ken about using a reading machine, and Ken makes several comments intended to irritate her. Discuss the reality of a patient's expressing the need for limits that show that the caregiver cares. See Clark, B. (1974). *Whose life is it anyway?* Chicago: Dramatic Publishing.

4. Discuss "The Depersonalization of Patients: A Profile Gleaned from Narratives" from the Readings section.

Session 6: **Tough Love**

Practice Hour

1. Discuss the reasons that compliance in therapy is important.

2. Why is limit-setting so often difficult?

3. Present the idea of limit-setting as another way of caring, which can be as valuable as more traditional nurturing.

4. Give examples of treatment situations that call for the therapist to set limits.

5. Discuss how methods used in setting limits vary with the situation, the client's cognitive/developmental level, and the client's emotional state.

6. Discuss levels of limit-setting (see handout).

Methods of Limit-Setting

1. Redirect or offer alternatives

   Example: "It's too late to start painting, but you could use markers if you want to."

2. Compromise

   Example: "Would you be willing to get your tub-transfer practice out of the way before working on the vase for your wife?"

3. Empathic refusal

   Example: "I understand that you are feeling distressed, but I must ask you to stay in occupational therapy for 10 more minutes."

4. Broken record

   Example: "No." "I am not comfortable with that." "I regret that it is not possible." "I cannot do that." "I am not interested." "I am firmly opposed to it."

5. Corrective feedback

   Example: "Mary, your outfit is attractive but too revealing for this work setting. What is your understanding of the dress code?"

6. Natural consequences

   Example: "When you hurry and slap on the paint, you have a lot of cleaning up to do." "When you do not come to therapy, I cannot sign your workman's compensation forms."

7. Imposed consequences

   Example: "When you curse in occupational therapy you must do a time-out." "If you do not complete your clean-up today, you will be unable to work on crafts tomorrow."

8. Commenting on patterns of behavior and analyzing causes and effects in an effort to find better alternatives

   Example: "I have noticed that you and I get along really well until about 10 minutes before the session ends, at which time you seem angry. What is that all about?"

Session 6: **Tough Love**

Role Play

Scenario A: Only You

Background: The 55-year-old patient has been living alone after the death of his spouse. He works as a machinist in an automobile factory and has been in weekly hand rehabilitation after a traumatic work-related injury. He has struggled with both the emotional trauma and the physical impairment. Through it all, the patient has confided in and relied on the occupational therapist who happens to be a Fieldwork II student.

Student therapist: Clinic policy states that socialization with patients is not allowed. You are very fond of this patient and are concerned about his lack of friends and family to lend support. You want to terminate this working relationship in a manner that is therapeutic and positive.

Session 6: **Tough Love**

Role Play

Scenario B: The Fashion Police

Background: The setting is a residential center designed to help persons with brain injuries make the transition from hospital-based rehabilitation into independent living arrangements. The client is a 25-year-old. Prior to a rock-climbing accident, the client was in medical school with a grade point average of 3.8 and an active social life. The patient's residual deficits include difficulty with manual dexterity, motor planning, and focusing on tasks.

Therapist: Your patient has arrived for the group outing to a moderately formal restaurant wearing torn gym shorts, a dirty sweatshirt with a logo that says, "Honk If You're Horny," and rubber sandals. You are compelled to help your client act appropriately in public and to preserve good public relations for your treatment center. You also need to reward your client's efforts to dress independently. Your client has 30 minutes to change before the group leaves.

Session 6: **Tough Love**

Role Play

Scenario C: Looking for Love

Background: The client is an older person of the opposite sex whose therapy includes massage and passive range of motion of the left upper extremity. This is your second of five sessions.

Therapist: You are a therapist at a hand therapy clinic. Your client persists in behaving in a manner that makes you very uncomfortable, and you want to help this client change the behavior while maintaining a therapeutic relationship. Begin by ranging and massaging your patient's affected arm and hand.

Session 6: **Tough Love**

Role Play

Scenario D: Tooling Around

Background: The patient is in the hospital for treatment of bipolar disorder, in a manic state. Yesterday, the patient became agitated during the occupational therapy session and gestured as if to hit a peer with a hammer, although no harm was done. The team has agreed to allow the patient to continue to attend the group with restrictions on the use of tools.

Therapist: You need to meet with the patient prior to the craft group this afternoon to discuss yesterday's incident and its consequences. You plan to discontinue the patient's access to tools until the patient demonstrates consistent self-control, but you may adjust your plan as you see fit. Remember that you represent the team and that you have a full menu of options for limit-setting.

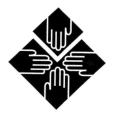

Session 7: **Making the Interview a Human Exchange**

Reflection Hour

1. Consider an excerpt (pp. 141–142) from H. H. Perlman, which is about an exchange between a young doctor and a woman who has gone to the hospital for treatment of an injured knee. The doctor misses the essential point of establishing rapport. See Perlman, H. H. (1979). *Relationship: The heart of helping people.* Chicago: University of Chicago Press.

   Discuss the following:

   • What is Perlman trying to say?

   • What might the young doctor have done/said differently?

   or

   • Have you had similar experiences either as a patient or caregiver?

   • What occasions in occupational therapy practice might present a similar challenge?

2. Consider whether you have ever had an encounter in health care during which you felt that your caregiver did not establish rapport with you. Discuss the experience.

3. Consider the challenge of trying to connect with the patient as a person while using a form or protocol for assessment or treatment. Discuss various interpretations of the challenge.

4. If some participants saw the challenge as an unresolved problem, discuss how the challenge might be met successfully.

Recommendation

Read "Using the Arts to Enhance Confluent Learning" from the Readings section.

Session 7: **Human Exchanges**

Practice Hour

The goal of these role plays is to practice simultaneously establishing a therapeutic relationship with the client, gathering needed information as outlined on a protocol, and probing for information that is relevant, but not specifically addressed on the protocol.

Session 7: **Human Exchanges**

Role Play

Scenario A: Developmental Dilemma

Background: The setting is an outpatient pediatric clinic in a large children's hospital. The client is Charley, a 5-year-old boy whose mother is worried about his development. The referring physician has reported some concern about possible family stress. The occupational therapist is meeting with the mother for an initial interview and developmental history.

Therapist: Use the Pediatric Initial Interview. You have been alerted that this mother seems to be more concerned about her child's development than is warranted, given that the doctor and teacher have been reassuring. Look for hidden agendas or causes for concern, and follow up on any hints of where the problem may lie.

Pediatric Initial Interview

Name _____

Date of Birth _____ Age _____

Parent's names _____

Developmental milestones (indicate approximate ages):

Eating solids _____ Sitting _____

Walking _____ Toilet training _____

First words _____ Phrases _____

Tricycle riding _____ Drawing _____

Writing name _____ Names letters _____

Play preferences _____

Peer relationships _____

Parents' concerns and goals _____

_____

Session 7: **Human Exchanges**

Role Play

Scenario B: The Difficult Delinquent

Background: The patient is a 13-year-old who has been hospitalized in a psychiatric unit. Child Protective Services sought the hospitalization after he ran away from several foster homes. Additional problem behaviors include stealing money from foster parents, threatening a teacher with a knife, promiscuity, and truancy from school.

Therapist: Use the Adolescent Initial Interview. Your primary goal is to initiate a therapeutic relationship with this very trouble adolescent and to calm any fears about being hospitalized. The unit nurses have described the patient as withdrawn and have had little luck in engaging the patient since his admission earlier that day.

Adolescent Initial Interview

Name _____

Date of Birth _____ Age _____

Parent's name(s) _____

School _____ Grade _____

Satisfaction with school performance _____

Extracurricular activities _____

Hobbies and sports interests _____

Friends and activities _____

Adult friends or relatives who provide support _____

Relationship with parents: Mother _____

Father _____

Reasons for hospitalization _____

Personal goals _____

Session 7: **Human Exchanges**

Role Play

Scenario C: Hot Potato

Background: The client is a special education teacher from a public school first grade. The teacher has had many years of experience and has a reputation for excellence. The occupational therapist and teacher are reviewing the teacher's responses on the Preassessment Checklist to try to define the needs of a student named Henry.

Therapist: You want to understand what is really troubling this teacher, who normally approaches challenges with a cool head. The teacher's responses on the checklist seem to be exaggerated.

Preassessment Checklist

Date: _____   Child's Name: Henry O.

Teacher/Therapist: Ms. Kiddo   Grade: First

Patterns noted in student's behavior	Never	Seldom	Occasionally	Often	Consistently
Copies letters & numbers legibly	X				
Spontaneously writes letters & numbers accurately	X				
Copies words and sentences legibly	X				
Reads at expected level for cognitive ability	X				
Works independently	X				
Completes all parts of worksheets	X				
Written work is neat	X				
Written work is generally correct	X				
Independently identifies errors in work	X				
Independently corrects errors in work	X				
Persists when tasks are challenging	X				
Seeks help appropriately	X				
Works at a reasonable pace	X				
Follows classroom routines and rules	X				
Cooperates with peers and adults	X				
Resolves interpersonal conflict effectively	X				
Expresses needs and wants effectively	X				
Remains task-focused despite typical distractions	X				
Considers consequences before acting	X				

Patterns noted in student's behavior	Never	Seldom	Occasionally	Often	Consistently
Regulates activity level to suit the situation	X				
Copes effectively with transitions and everyday stresses	X				
Holds pencil in a mature manor	X				
Cuts effectively	X				
Learns new motor tasks given opportunity to practice	X				

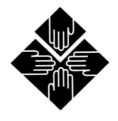

Session 8: **Whose Life Is It Anyway?**

Reflection Hour

1. Consider the poem "Some Other Day." The poem is about an occupational therapist's exchange with an older woman. See McClay, E. (1987, March). Green Winter: Celebration of old age. *Reader's Digest*, pp. 106–109.

    Discuss the following:

    - What has happened in this exchange?
    - What went wrong?
    - What actions might have been taken instead?
    - What activities might have been therapeutic for this woman?
    - Whose treatment plan is it anyway?

2. Consider an excerpt (pp. 166–167) from J. Heller and S. Vogel that describes Heller's experience with Guillain-Barré syndrome and occupational therapy. Discuss the similarities and differences between Heller's experience with therapy that did not consider his needs and the story of the older woman in the poem "Some Other Day." See Heller, J., & Vogel, S. (1986). *No laughing matter.* New York: Avon Books.

3. Discuss "Using the Arts to Enhance Confluent Learning" from the Readings section. Consider any connections that you can make with today's theme.

Options and Alternatives

Consider a passage (pp. 228–230) from Ken Kesey's novel, which relates an incident between the aides and patient George Sefelt. It is an extreme illustration of a treatment plan implemented against the patient's will. Discuss the feelings that patients have when they are excluded from making decisions about their treatment. See Kesey, K. (1962). *One flew over the cuckoo's nest.* New York: Signet Books.

Recommendation

Read "The Fullness of Empathy: Reflections and Illustrations" from the Readings section.

Session 8: **Whose Life Is It Anyway?**

Practice Hour

1. Discuss intervention as a collaborative process.

    - Historically, medicine has been viewed as an interaction involving a practitioner doing something to or for a patient for the patient's good.

    - Do you think this perspective is a valid one today?

    - Does the idea of the patient as a passive recipient fit with the current philosophy and practice of occupational therapy?

2. What kinds of factors could make sharing information or collaboration with a patient or a patient's family especially challenging?

Session 8: **Whose Life Is It Anyway?**

Role Play

Scenario A: Independent Elder

Background: Mrs. Henry is a 73-year-old widow who lives alone in a small house in a lower income section of Chicago. She has two daughters who live in Chicago and a son who lives in Los Angeles. Mrs. Henry had a right CVA 3 days ago and is moving into a rehabilitation unit of the hospital. She is expected to be discharged to her home and the care of her daughters after 2 weeks. She has seen the occupational therapist for two evaluation sessions, and the following treatment plan is a provisional draft that needs to be reviewed with Mrs. Henry prior to its implementation.

Therapist: Use Mrs. Henry's treatment plan on the following page. You feel strongly that for safety reasons Mrs. Henry will need daily assistance from family members or a home health nurse or therapist during her first weeks at home. You recognize that some of her emotional reactions are related to neurological effects of the CVA and that they may change later as she progresses physiologically. You also recognize that, as reported by her family, Mrs. Henry has always been the family leader and is fiercely independent. You need to gain Mrs. Henry's confidence and to get her started in treatment as soon as possible.

Session 8: **Whose Life Is It Anyway?**

Role Play

Scenario A: Independent Elder   Treatment Plan: Mrs. Henry (1/5/97)

Assets: Walks with quad cane
            Motivated to return home
            Supportive family

Limitations: Needs moderate assistance for dressing
                Spatial memory impairment
                Inconsistent safety awareness

Discharge Plan: Return to home with intermittent supervision

Long-term goal

Mrs. Henry will be independent in dressing.

Current status

Needs assistance to don slacks, socks, undergarments, and shirts.

Short-term goals

• Will have passive range of motion to 110 degrees flexion of right shoulder by 1/15.

• Will learn adaptive dressing techniques by 1/20.

• Will dress independently in front-buttoning shirts and pull-on pants or skirts by 1/25.

Long-term goal

Mrs. Henry will navigate independently in familiar settings without becoming lost.

Current status:

Is unable to locate any personal items in her room or to find work areas within the unit.

Short-term goals

• Will independently locate her personal belongings without trial-and-error 75% of the time by 1/10.

• Will independently find her way to all work areas within the rehabilitation unit by 1/15.

• Will independently find her way around her home and neighborhood by discharge.

Long-term goal

Mrs. Henry will adhere to safety precautions at home and in the community and will obtain assistance as needed.

Current status

Forgets to turn off grooming and kitchen appliances 1 to 3 times per day and often refuses assistance when having difficulty.

Short-term goals

- Will identify safety hazards in simulated kitchen and bathroom settings with 100% accuracy by 1/10.

- Will spontaneously turn off appliances 100% of the time by 1/10.

- Will request and accept assistance as needed by 1/15.

Session 8: **Whose Life Is It Anyway?**

Role Play

Scenario B: Caustic College Student

Background: Connie is a 25-year-old college student who is completing her last semester of a masters degree in quantum physics. She has been diagnosed with major recurrent depression since she was 18, and is in a day treatment program following a 1-week hospitalization after a suicide attempt. She has completed an occupational therapy evaluation and needs to hear the results and recommendations. Connie and the therapist have established a working relationship based on mutual liking and respect, but Connie has consistently resisted viewing herself as a part of the larger client group.

Therapist: You have assessed Connie with a standardized self-concept scale and observations of task performance with macramé and a simple cooking activity. You have also observed her social behavior with other clients and with you. Your assessment consists of the following:

Self-Concept Scale Profile

Social relations:	10th percentile
Health/wellness:	16th percentile
Physical appearance and skills:	20th percentile
Intelligence:	84th percentile
Academic or work performance:	70th percentile
Leisure performance:	4th percentile
Optimism scale:	9th percentile

Strengths: Intelligence, quality, and skills related to task performance and family support.

Limitations: Low-self-esteem, underdeveloped awareness of emotions, poor communication skills (often sarcastic), few friends or social supports, and poor balance of work and leisure.

Your recommendations include 3 half-days of occupational therapy per week including assertiveness training, stress management, and leisure skills development groups.

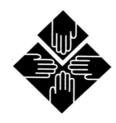

Session 9: **What It Means to Be a Colleague**

Reflection Hour

1. The focus of the course is now shifting to interpersonal skills, empathy, and the use of self in terms of participants' relationships with colleagues.

2. Respond to the question "Who [in various day-to-day settings] will my colleagues be?" or "Who are my colleagues?"

3. The fable is a literary device through which authors make statements about human nature by using animals as primary characters.

   • Consider James Thurber's "The Very Proper Gander." See Thurber, J. (1940). *Fables for our times*. New York: Harper Brothers. Discuss the relevance of the fable to practice among colleagues. Anticipate problematic situations that may occur in practice or discuss past relevant experiences that come to mind after hearing the fable.

   • Consider James Thurber's "The Fairly Intelligent Fly." See Thurber, J. (1940). *Fables for our times*. New York: Harper Brothers. Discuss this fable's relevance to practice among colleagues. Anticipate problematic situations or discuss relevant experiences.

4. Discuss 'The Fullness of Empathy: Reflection and Illustrations" from the Readings section.

Session 9: **What It Means to Be a Colleague**

Practice Hour

1. *Discussion question*: When do occupational therapists need to be negotiators or mediators in conflict resolution with clients and with colleagues?

2. Review the following references on negotiation. See Fisher, R., & Ury, W. (1991). *Getting to yes: Negotiating agreement without giving in*. New York: Penguin; Fisher, R., & Brown, S. (1988). *Getting together: Building relationships as we negotiate*. New York: Penguin.

3. Consider the basic steps in resolving conflict:

   • Identify your true goals. Think about specific behaviors.

      1. Prioritize. Know what you can afford to give up.

      2. Formulate alternative ideas regarding how needs may be met.

   • Separate the problem from the person.

      1. The primary goal is development of the working relationship.

      2. The secondary goal is resolution of the issues.

   • Strive to understand the goals and concerns of others.

      1. Ask and listen.

      2. Operate with the belief that disagreement is okay, Approval is not necessary for a positive working relationship, and Shared values are not a prerequisite for a positive working relationship.

   • Avoid "we"/"they" thinking and speaking and work toward "we" thinking.

      1. Look beyond stereotypes—active listening is helpful for this.

      2. Respect and value the point of view of others and their right to have another perspective.

      3. Respect and use organization and social structure.

      4. Do not try to force or "buy" the relationship. Coercion may be effective in the short run, but costly in the long run.

An Unconditionally Constructive Strategy

"Do only those things that are both good for the relationship and good for us, whether or not they reciprocate."

Rationality: Even if they are acting emotionally, balance emotions with reason.

Understanding: Even if they misunderstand, try to understand them.

Communication: Even if they are not listening, consult them before deciding on matters that affect them.

Reliability: Even if they are trying to deceive us, neither trust them nor deceive them. Be reliable.

Noncoercive Modes of Influence: Even if they are trying to coerce us, neither yield to that coercion nor try to coerce them. Be open to persuasion and try to persuade them.

Acceptance: Even if they reject us and our concerns as unworthy of their consideration, accept them as worthy of our consideration, care about them, and be open to learning from them.

From Fisher, R., & Brown, S. (1988). *Getting together: Building relationships as we negotiate.* New York: Penguin. Reprinted with permission.

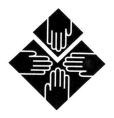

Session 10: **Is There Room for Compromise?**

Reflection Hour

1. Consider compromises you could suggest in the following situation: Person A wants a triangle, but Person B wants a circle.

2. Briefly discuss responses as they relate to individual definitions of the term *compromise*. Discuss similarities and differences in views.

3. Consider the children's story *The giving tree.* To what extent has compromise been portrayed? See Silverstein, S. (1964). *The giving tree.* New York: Harper & Row.

   • What has the tree given? What has the tree gotten?

   • What has the boy given? What has the boy gotten?

   • Is there a balance or mutual satisfaction in the exchange?

   • Must compromise be an equal give and take?

   • What are the implications of this portrayal of compromise for practice among colleagues?

4. Consider a situation in which you chose to compromise. Discuss the experience.

Recommendation

Read "Art: An Occupation with Promise for Developing Empathy" in the Readings section.

Session 10: **Is There Room for Compromise?**

Role Play

Scenario A: Delicate Matters

Background: An occupational therapist who has just started working in a skilled nursing facility is reviewing the caseload. Upon looking over the charts and meeting the patients, the therapist discovers that two comatose patients have been prescribed an inappropriate daily-living training regime. The occupational therapist approaches the supervisor, an administrator, about the matter.

Occupational Therapist: You have a strong commitment to providing the most appropriate care to each patient and avoiding inaccurate documentation or unnecessary costs for the patients or their funders. You believe that the patients in question should have weekly monitor checks, with an aide providing daily range-of-motion and sensory stimulation programs.

Session 10: **Is There Room for Compromise?**

Role Play

Scenario B: Fire and Ice

Background: Two experienced occupational therapists have recently started working together to start up the occupation theory component of a day treatment program for adolescents with chemical dependency and conduct disorders. They are dismayed to find that their clinical styles do not mesh easily, as exemplified by this incident: An adolescent client became angry when Therapist A told him that he could not paint gang symbols on a T-shirt. The client responded by throwing the shirt into a trash can and cursing the therapist. The therapist responded by saying, "It's really hard for you to accept limits on what you can do on your project. What is it that makes you feel so bad about that?" They went on to discuss the incident, which led to talking about how the client feels at home when his parents use humiliation and threats to control him.

Therapist B: You come from a varied background that includes 10 years in inpatient psychiatry. You are most comfortable with an insight-oriented approach in therapy. You feel very good about your interaction with the difficult client today, as your primary goal is for him to understand and express his feelings. However, you can see that your cotherapist is now angry.

Session 10: **Is There Room for Compromise?**

Role Play

Scenario C: Showdown at the OK Corral

Background: The OK Care Center is a residential facility for geriatric patients who need skilled care. The occupational therapist (who has been at "OK" for 1 month) is meeting with the head nurse (who has been at "OK" for 25 years) to discuss mealtime management. The therapist has observed that many residents who could be eating independently or with moderate assistance are being fed pureed food in their rooms.

Therapist: You are disturbed to see the isolation and infantilization that these older people have to endure at mealtimes. You feel that eating should be a pleasant social experience and that food should provide satisfying tastes and textures. You have the sense that the staff members are not aware of the latest techniques for helping people with cognitive and sensorimotor deficits relearn how to feed themselves and eat table foods safely. You have recently completed a continuing education course on this topic and are eager to try out new adaptive equipment and teaching methods. To do so, you will need the cooperation of the nursing staff.

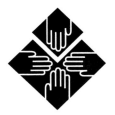

Session 11: **Supervision—Taking It**

Reflection Hour

1. Discussion questions: "Who might your supervisors be?" or "Who are your supervisors?"

2. Reflect on the kind of supervisory situation or input that has been (or may be) most difficult for you to deal with.

3. Discuss the various meanings of the phrase *taking supervision*.

   • What does the phrase mean in its positive or best sense? When is taking supervision easy to do?

   • What does the phrase mean in its negative or worst sense? What circumstances make supervision hard to take?

4. Consider an excerpt from John Pekkanen (pp. 24–25). See Pekkanen, J. (1981). *M.D.: Doctors talk about themselves*. New York: Dell. Discuss the nature and quality of the supervisory exchange.

5. Consider an exchange from Joanne Greenberg's account (see pp. 92–94). A psychiatric aide named McPherson gives a patient, Deborah, corrective feedback on her behavior toward an abusive aide. Discuss the nature and quality of the exchange. See Greenberg, J. (as Green, H.) (1964). *I never promised you a rose garden*. New York: Holt, Rinehart & Winston.

6. Discuss "Art: An Occupation With Promise for Developing Empathy" from the Readings section. Consider to what extent individuals need to empathize during supervision.

Session 11: **Supervision—Taking It**

Practice Hour

Dealing with Supervision

Discuss the concept of "supervision".

Give an example of a time that you have experienced corrective feedback (which is helpful) or criticism (which is often designed to cause pain).

Responses to corrective feedback or criticism may include:

Negative inquiry: an active listening response involving paraphrasing and seeking clarification in a nondefensive manner. (See accompanying dialog.)

"I statements": an assertive communication response in which the listener shares his reactions in a responsible and nonblaming style. Example: "I feel uncomfortable when I am corrected in front of the patients.", rather than, "You make me feel like a jerk when you correct me in front of others."

Cognitive coping messages: internal dialog with oneself to facilitate positive and rational thinking during stressful situations. Examples: "I am here to learn, and this feedback will help me grow."; "I've made a mistake, but I will learn from this and go on to do well."; "She's had a bad day and needs to blow off steam right now."

Fogging: a last resort measure when one is quite certain that the criticism being offered is abusive in nature, and is of little value to one's development. (See accompanying dialog.)

Session 11: **Supervision—Taking It**

Practice Hour
Negative Inquiry Example Dialogue

Felix: "This place looks like a pig sty!"

Oscar: "What bothers you about it?"

Felix: "Just look at it—dirty dishes all over the place. It stinks!"

Oscar: "So you think I need to wash the dishes more often. Is there anything else?"

Felix: "I can't even see the floor for all of the dirty clothes strewn around. Do you ever do your laundry?"

Oscar: "Is it pretty much the clothes on the floor that bothers you, or the ones on the sofa and chairs, too?"

Felix: "*All* of it! Have you always been such a slob?"

Oscar: "Are the dishes and clothes the main concerns, or are there other things that I could work on?"

Felix: "Your sense of decor seems to be early rummage sale; where did you find this lamp— in a haunted house?"

Oscar: "Do you think that it's the shade that's wrong, or what?"

Felix: "No, I'd keep the shade and toss the rest of it!"

Oscar: "So the shade is acceptable, but the lamp is unattractive?"

Felix: "That's right."

Oscar: "So, if I work on the dishes, the laundry, and the lamp, would there be any other improvements that you would recommend?"

Felix: "I guess not."

Oscar: "Thanks for your ideas. I appreciate your concern."

Session 11: **Supervision—Taking It**

Practice Hour
"Fogging" Dialogue

Prying Pip: "I've heard there's some interesting goings-on in your department. Is it true that your boss is about to get fired?"

Peaceful Pat: "I really couldn't say."

Prying Pip: "Oh, come on, Pat. You and I go way back."

Peaceful Pat: "Yes, we've known each other for quite awhile."

Prying Pip: "So dish some dirt with me, pal! I've heard he got caught with his hand in the cookie jar."

Peaceful Pat: "There are certainly many rumors."

Prying Pip: "I've also been hearing about Dr. Goodbar and Miss Fanny. Were they really caught in the linen closet?"

Peaceful Pat: "Some people say so."

Prying Pip: "And what about that patient up on the third floor, the one that supposedly thinks he's a reincarnated tree? Is it true that he has a bird in his beard?"

Peaceful Pat: "I hadn't heard that."

Prying Pip: "And what's this I hear about you and that new therapist in Burns? Is it true blondes have more fun?"

Peaceful Pat: "Oh, Pip, you're such a tease!"

Prying Pip: "You should stop being such a hermit and get out more. Why not take up mud wrestling? It's done wonders for me!"

Peaceful Pat: "I'll have to give it some thought."

Prying Pip: "Well, gotta go! You're always a wealth of juicy information!"

Peaceful Pat: "Good bye!"

Session 11: **Supervision: Taking It**

Role Play

Scenario A: A petunia in an onion patch

Background: The setting is a rehabilitation center where the philosophy is oriented toward physical concerns. This morning Mrs. Grant, who had a CVA 2 weeks ago, began to cry about 5 minutes into the session while stacking cones. The student therapist (OTS) discontinued the activity and sat down with her. The OTS spent the next 20 minutes listening as Mrs. Grant expressed feelings that ranged from fear to anger. The session ended with Mrs. Grant appearing refreshed and relaxed and agreeing to make cookies for her grandson in the OT kitchen the next day.

Supervisee: You are using the skills and values that were taught at your progressive and holistically-oriented OT school, and feel that your choices are clinically sound. However, you have another month to go in this placement, and do not stand much chance of changing your supervisor's philosophy. Work to convey a willingness to honor your supervisor's perspective while also honoring your contract with Mrs. G.

Session 11: **Supervision—Taking It**

Role Play

Scenario B: Wild in the streets

Background: The setting is a day hospital for adolescent mental health clients. The OTS has just completed a craft group that did not turn out as well as planned. The project involved free-form painting of T shirts. During the session things got somewhat out of control: shirts were decorated with rude and provocative slogans, paint was spilled on upholstered chairs, and the teens were sassy. The OTS and supervisor are debriefing.

OTS: You know that this session has not been your best. Use negative inquiry to learn how you can improve.

Session 11: **Supervision: Taking It**

Role Play

Scenario C: Changing Times

Background: The new staff OT and supervisor attended team rounds together this morning for the first time. The supervisor has been at this rehabilitation center for 20 years. The staff OT has been at the facility for three weeks, and has quickly developed a warm working relationship with the rest of the treatment team. During the meeting the OT volunteered evaluation and treatment information, which was well received by the group.

Staff OT: You feel good about the way rounds went today. You're especially pleased that Mr. Jones's discharge to a nursing facility has been postponed, as you feel optimistic that he will improve rapidly enough to go home within the next week. (Similar patients whom you have treated have shown such patterns of improvement in therapy.)

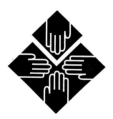

Session 12: **Supervision—Giving It**

Reflection Hour

1. Recall from Session 11 the kind of exchange between a supervisor and supervisee that would be easy to take.

2. Discuss

   • Must a supervisor *like* every supervisee?

   • What qualities about the supervisory exchange that you have identified above might be difficult to implement or to control?

   • What other situations might make giving supervision difficult?

3. Consider an excerpt from Clark (pp. 49–51). Dr. Emerson and Dr. Scott disagree on a matter of patient care. See Clark, B. (1974). *Whose life is it anyway?* Chicago: Dramatic Publishing.

4. Consider an exchange from Kesey's work (pp. 86–89) in which the big nurse chastises the aides (Washington and Williams) as she deals with the patient McMurphy's complaint. Discuss the specific behaviors that are troublesome in this exchange. See Kesey, K. (1962). *One flew over the cuckoo's nest.* New York: Signet.

5. Share a personal story or experience that illustrates supervision's being given well or not so well.

Session 12: **Supervision—Giving It**

Practice Hour

1. Discuss the situations in which you will find yourself responsible for providing supervision.

2. Briefly review the variety of techniques for limit-setting that were covered in Session 6, Tough Love. Which of these would work best with supervisees?

Session 12: **Supervision—Giving It**

Role Play

Scenario A: Too Many Irons

Background: The setting is a skilled nursing facility where patients are often seen in groups of 6 to 12. The patient caseload per therapist has doubled in the past 6 months because of decreases in staff and increases in the patient population, and all are feeling the pinch. The occupational therapy supervisor (who has been there 1 month) learned this morning that a certified occupational therapy assistant (COTA) supervisee, the supervisor's senior by 15 years, has been leaving the craft group patients alone for 15 to 20 minutes during each session to photocopy the supervisor's paperwork. The patients are charged for a full hour of therapy.

Supervisor: You are concerned for the following reasons: patient safety, professional liability (the COTA's, yours, and the institution's), the ethics of charging for therapy when no therapist is present, the COTA's apparent poor judgment about prioritizing assignments and managing time, and the COTA's unwillingness to approach you about her difficulty with managing the workload.

Session 12: **Supervision—Giving It**

Role Play

Scenario B: White Rabbit Syndrome

Background: The setting is a busy inpatient rehabilitation center. The occupational therapist supervisor and treatment team have been repeatedly annoyed and inconvenienced when the occupational therapy field work student, who has been at this setting for 3 weeks, has been consistently 5 to 15 minutes late for meetings and supervision sessions. Punctuality and formality are strong values in this particular facility.

Supervisor: Your student initially seemed very bright and well prepared, but you have noticed an air of preoccupation and a tendency to overextend herself. You want to provide enough guidance to keep things safe and productive but do not believe in "spoon feeding." Try to give feedback and explore the possible causes of the difficulties.

Session 12: **Supervision—Giving It**

Role Play

Scenario C: The Fashion Police

Background: A student has arrived for the first day of preceptorship at a church-affiliated hospital occupational therapy clinic wearing black leather from head to toe, very strong cologne, and a punk hairstyle. To top it off, the student is loudly snapping and chewing a large piece of gum.

Supervisor: You want this student to go home and return looking more suitable for work before anyone else sees her. You also want to start off your relationship in a positive manner.

Session 12: **Supervision—Giving It**

Role Play

Scenario D: Now You See Them—Now You Don't!

Background: The setting is a public school where a second occupational therapist has recently joined the special education department. The supervising occupational therapist has worked diligently to convince school administrators and teachers that the students with behavior disorders can benefit from occupational therapy services, and she has been allowed to start such a group in one of the schools. The new occupational therapist, who recently began working with this group, discharged all of the children from occupational therapy after only 3 weeks, saying that they had reached maximum benefit.

Supervisor: You are extremely upset that this new therapist has discontinued services that you think are needed, and that she has harmed your credibility with the rest of the team. You want to understand the therapist's rationale for this decision and to impress upon the therapist that you must approve any decisions about discontinuation of services before the decisions are made public.

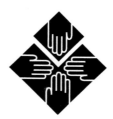

Session 13: **Saying No and Saving Face**

Reflection Hour

1. Consider a passage from Reiser and Schroder (see pp. 3–10). The scenario depicts an exchange among a medical student, a respiratory therapist, and a physician. Dr. Gellman sets limits on the respiratory therapist. See Reiser, D., & Schroder, A. K. (1975). *Patient interviewing: The human dimension.* San Francisco: Institute for the study of Humanistic Medicine. Then consider a segment (pp. 238–239) from Rebeta-Burditt, where Cassie calls her Alcoholics Anonymous sponsor who says no to her request. See Rebeta-Burditt, J. (1977). *The cracker factory.* New York: Bantam Books. Discuss these segments in terms of the manner in which limits were or were not set and face was or was not saved.

2. Review a sampling of three or four cartoons that illustrate various ways of saying no. The following are excellent sources. See Callahan, J. (1991). *Digesting the child within.* New York: Morrow. See Kliban, B. (1986). *The biggest tongue in Tunisia.* New York: Penguin. See Larsen, G. (1986, 1988). *The far side gallery.* Kansas City, MO: Andrews and McNeel. Discuss the following questions in pairs:

   • What does it mean to "say no and save face?"

   • What does an exchange look like in which one "loses face" compared with one in which one "saves face?"

   • What requests or situations make it hard for you to say no? (When will it be hardest for you to say no to colleagues or supervisor in practice?)

3. Present your responses to the group, commenting on similarities and differences in remarks.

4. Discuss the benefits of saying no.

Session 13: **Saying No and Saving Face**

Practice Hour

1. Discuss types of situations that might require limit-setting with peers or superiors at work. Give an example from your experience.

2. Briefly review limit-setting techniques from Session 6. Discuss which techniques would be most likely to work best with peers and supervisors.

3. After role playing, assign roles for next week's all-class role play in a school team meeting situation. Bring any props that you would like. Think about your role and opinions on issues raised by the case.

Session 13: **Saying No and Saving Face**

Role Play

Scenario A: Looking for Dr. Goodbar

Background: The setting is a fast-paced occupational therapy practice that specializes in out-patient work evaluation and treatment, and the "players" are staff occupational therapists. The group values teamwork, quality care, and productivity. This is the third time this month that a request like this has occurred.

Therapist: You have left the hour between 4 and 5 o'clock to catch up on paperwork and are pleased with yourself for meeting a personal goal to leave work on time tonight. You have no special plans after work but have been feeling overextended and wish to avoid burnout.

Session 13: **Saying No and Saving Face**

Role Play

Scenario B: East Meets West

Background: The setting is a children's psychiatric day treatment facility. Historically, there has ben disagreement about whether occupational therapy should be used as a reward for appropriate behavior. The occupational therapists and the program director have asked that occupational therapy be considered as a therapy, not a reinforcement. Not all members of the team agree with this new policy. The occupational therapist has arrived in the unit to bring 8-year-old Mikey to occupational therapy and is speaking with a teacher colleague.

Therapist: You think that using occupational therapy as a reward results in withholding needed therapy from students whose misbehavior is symptomatic of their mental health problems. This reduces occupational therapy to "playtime" in the eyes of the rest of the team. You also know that you and the teacher will need to work together. It may be possible to negotiate (for example, offer to see Mikey in the classroom, rather than in the usual clinic group). Find out if the teacher knows about the new policy.

Session 13: **Saying No and Saving Face**

Role Play

Scenario C: Just Ducky!

Background: The setting is an outpatient rehabilitation clinic that specializes in neurodevelopmental therapies. The occupational therapy supervisor is a renowned specialist who has recently returned from a lengthy sabbatical on a remote Caribbean island where the therapist lived with the natives and developed an interest in spirituality and alternative healing practices.

Therapist: You are conservative by nature and feel most comfortable in a traditional medical environment. You do not wish to engage in professional practices that are unresearched and highly controversial, yet you wish to remain employed at this facility for at least another year. You have a good reputation as an effective therapist.

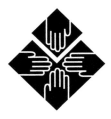

Session 14: **Sharing the Plan**

Reflection Hour

1. Consider the opportunity that reflection provides to think through problematic inter-personal situations. Discuss the merits of working through such situations before they occur. Think of a problem situation for the group to consider:

   What if I plan/try to _____ but a colleague _____.

   Describe some strategy learned in this course that might be helpful in resolving the problematic situations described.

2. Discuss the notion of patient advocacy with colleagues:

   • Consider a passage (pp. 103–106) from Joanne Greenberg in *I never promised you a rose garden*.

   • Discuss who demonstrated advocacy and how Dr. Furii might have become an advocate without compromising her relationship with the institution? See Greenberg, J. (1964).

Recommendation

To prepare for the final written assignment, read "The Patient–Therapist Relationship: Beliefs that Shape Care" and "Now That We Have Managed Care, Shall We Inspire It?" from the Readings section.

Session 14: **Sharing the Plan**

Practice Hour

Scenario: Too Many Cooks?

Cast of Characters:

Joe Student: 17-year-old high school junior with severe cerebral palsy

Madge Student: Joe's mother

Pete Student: Joe's father

Mr. or Ms. English: Writing teacher

Mr. or Ms. Work: Vocational training specialist for district

Mr. or Ms. Vowel: Speech therapist

Mr. or Ms. Function: Occupational therapist for district

Mr. or Ms. Boss: Special education administrator

Background: The setting is a public high school individualized educational program (IEP) meeting for Joe Student, a 17-year-old junior who has an IQ of 130 and severe cerebral palsy. Joe gets around with an electric wheelchair and has an attendant who has been hired by the school to assist him and two other students with personal care and eating. Although his speech is unintelligible, Joe has been attending regular high school courses, including honors math and science. He is able to complete written work with a word processor and an adapted keyboard and communicates basic needs and wants with a picture communication board. This is an end-of-year meeting to make critical decisions about Joe's senior year, during which he must prepare for life after high school. Each person at the meeting should strive to have his or her viewpoints heard and understood, while respecting the rights and views of the others.

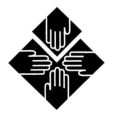

Session 15: **Your Turn**

Reflection Hour

Take an opportunity to reflect on and evaluate the experience of the course, given more specific written guidelines from the facilitator.

Recommendation

Read "Now That We Have Managed Care, Shall We Inspire it?" and "The Patient–Therapist Relationship: Beliefs That Shape Care" from the Readings section.

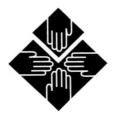

V. Readings

BRIEF OR NEW

Interpersonal Skills for Practice: An Elective Course

Suzanne M. Peloquin,
Debora A. Davidson

Key Words: professional–patient relations •
teaching methods

Suzanne M. Peloquin, PhD, OTR, is Assistant Professor, Department of Occupational Therapy, School of Allied Health Sciences, The University of Texas Medical Branch, Galveston, Texas. (Mailing address: 4400 Ursuline #180, Galveston, Texas 77550)

Debora A. Davidson, MS, OTR, is Assistant Professor, Department of Occupational Therapy, School of Allied Health Sciences, The University of Texas Medical Branch, Galveston, Texas.

This article was accepted for publication August 1, 1992.

This past year, faculty at the School of Allied Health Sciences of the University of Texas Medical Branch at Galveston offered an elective course to enhance student preparedness to face the interpersonal challenges that are apt to occur in practice. One catalyst for the development of this course was a letter from a student that read in part: "It has been a great challenge trying to apply everything from books to real life situations. The books don't teach you how to react when the patient's finger starts to bleed in treatment or how to comfort your patient when she starts to cry during an evaluation." The challenge of how to *be* in practice, how to be both personal and professional, is one that each student will ultimately face. And, as Mosey said, the challenge is very much an individual one: "Each student brings to her initial education a collection of memories regarding personal experiences and interaction with the self, other individuals, and the nonhuman environment. Each student has varying degrees of inner security, knowledge of self, and self-acceptance" (1981, p. 25). The call for such preparedness rests on two fundamental and traditional concepts known more currently as the art of practice and the therapeutic use of self. If students are to practice the art of occupational therapy, and if they are to use themselves therapeutically, they must learn to do so.

Aims of the Course

The occupational therapy curriculum at The University of Texas Medical Branch offers several opportunities to learn or review concepts and strategies related to the interpersonal aspects of practice. Explored during both the lecture and lab formats of two basic courses required early in the junior year, these concepts include

- conscious use of self
- values clarification
- therapeutic use of self
- nonverbal communication skills
- verbal communication skills such as
  active listening
  responding styles
  the understanding response
  reflecting and paraphrasing
  benefits of self-disclosure
  assertive behavior
  use of humor
- sharing information about treatment procedures
- using language that the patient can understand
- individual differences in therapist and patient styles
- interviewing skills
- open-ended versus close-ended questions
- collaborating with the patient
- treatment planning around patient goals
- occupational therapy groups

- limit-setting and troubleshooting strategies
- member roles in groups
- leader roles
- process versus content issues

The newly developed elective aims to supplement what students have already learned, to offer them an additional opportunity to enhance their sense of readiness for practice. Named "Interpersonal Skills for Practice," the course embodies a fundamental belief, articulated by Plum (1981), that rather than being just a set of skills, "communication is as rich, and sometimes as puzzling, as the human condition itself" (p. 18). Plum stated that, if practitioners are to demonstrate care, they must place understanding at the heart of personal communication. He argued:

> It is possible to help people improve the sensitivity and accuracy with which they perceive other people's messages, to provide them with conceptual tools to help them understand other people, and to aid them in enlarging their imaginative capacities so that they can see the world from other people's perspectives. (p. 15)

This course aims at the fundament of personal communication by offering opportunities to reflect about, experience, and respond to life-like situations. Four aspects of learning seem critical to the development of empathy: tuning in to oneself, expressing oneself, tuning in to others, and responding to others (Tubesing & Tubesing, 1973). These four functions constitute the four overarching goals of this elective.

Description of the Course

The elective offers students two academic credits and consists of a two-hour session held weekly. The class membership consists of students in their second year of enrollment in the program, not to exceed a group of 14. One hour of the class involves a discussion of phenomenological narratives; the second hour consists of role-play activities. Each instructor organizes and leads one of the two hours and co-leads the second. The course description promises that students will have an opportunity to: (a) explore effective ways of communicating with patients and colleagues, (b) identify various components and styles of communication, (c) analyze personal styles of communication, (d) describe the application of various communication techniques in therapeutic and collegial relationships, (e) develop a repertoire of effective communication skills that are applicable to a variety of challenging interpersonal situations, and (f) apply concepts and techniques used in communication skills treatment.

At the first meeting, students receive the following course schedule that orients them to the topics that will constitute their weekly focus:

- Week 1: Becoming Personal and Professional
- Week 2: The Therapeutic Use of Self
- Week 3: Active Listening
- Week 4: Non-Verbal Communication
- Week 5: The Power of Feelings
- Week 6: Caring Enough to Set Limits. Tough Love
- Week 7: Making the Interview a Human Exchange
- Week 8: Whose Life is it Anyway?
- Week 9: What It Means to be a Colleague
- Week 10: Is There Room for Compromise?
- Week 11: Supervision: Taking It
- Week 12: Supervision: Giving It
- Week 13: Saying No and Saving Face
- Week 14: Sharing the Plan

During the first meeting, students hear the views of Plum (1981) and Tubesing and Tubesing (1973) about empathy and the heart of communication, to ensure that they understand that the course aims to develop their abilities to reflect, empathize, and respond.

Strategies and Assignments: A Sampling

During the first hour of the class on Active Listening, an instructor might begin with an excerpt from a reading such as the poem "Some Other Day" (Maclay, 1977).

> Preserve me from the occupational therapist, God
> She means well, but I'm too busy to make baskets.
> I want to relive a day in July when Sam and I went berrying.
> I was eighteen, my hair was long and thick and I braided it and
>   wound it round my head so it wouldn't get caught on the briars.
> But when we sat in the shade to rest I unpinned it and it came
>   tumbling down.
> And Sam proposed.
> I suppose it wasn't fair to use my hair to make him fall in love
>   with me but it turned out to be a good marriage. . .
> Oh, here she comes, the therapist, with scissors and paste.
> "Would I like to try decoupage?"
> "No" I say, "I haven't got time."
> "Nonsense," she says, "You're going to live a long, long time."
> That's not what I mean. I mean that all my life I've been doing
>   things for people, with people. I have to catch up on my
>   thinking and feeling.
> About Sam's death, for one thing.
> Close to the end, I asked if there was anything I could do. . .
> He said, "Yes, unpin your hair."
> I said, "Oh, Sam, it's so thin now and gray,"
> "Please," he said, "Unpin it anyway."
> I did and he reached out his hand — the skin transparent, I could see
>   the blue veins — and stroked my hair.
> If I close my eyes, I can feel it, Sam.
> "Please open your eyes," the therapist says;
> "You don't want to sleep the day away,"
> She wants to know what I used to do,
> Knit? Crochet?
> Yes, I did those things, and cooked and cleaned, and raised five
>   children and had things happen to me.
> Beautiful things, terrible things.
> I need to think about them, arrange them on the shelves of my
>   mind.
> The therapist is showing me glittery beads.
> She asks if I might like to make jewelry.
> She's a dear child and means well,
> So I tell her I might.
> Some other day. (pp. 107–8)

After the reading, these questions generate much discussion and reflection: (a) Did this therapist listen? (b) What did the therapist not hear? (c) How did an occupational therapy protocol get in the way? (d) What occupation might have held therapeutic value for this woman? (e) Respond differently to this woman as she says to you, "No, I haven't got time." (f) Respond to her when she says "Some other day."

Other phenomenological narratives can stimulate similar discussion (for a bibliography, see suggested readings). Because fictional stories also exemplify the powerful exchanges that occur in health care practice, readers may want to refer to earlier bibliographies published in this journal (Peloquin, 1989, 1990).

A discussion of such narratives sets the stage for introducing the various weekly themes. Each theme is then explored more deeply as students role-play their responses to related situations that they might encounter in practice. A sampling of some of these situations includes the following:

> A patient says to you, the occupational therapist: "I hate you and I'll never come to OT again!" or "You're not going to make me do that are you? I feel lousy today." Respond. (Week 5: The Power of Feelings)

> You and I are peers who work together with an adolescent population. My style is permissive and interpretive. Yours is behavioral and more restrained. I keep letting patients break clinic rules of good manners, cleaning up after each session, and doing activities according to the established protocol. You are hoping to achieve better co-therapy. How will you approach me? What will you say? (Week 10: Is There Room For Compromise?)

> A physical therapist says to you, the occupational therapist: "You know, Mr. Saunders needs gait training more than work on crafts at this point. Can I see him for a half-hour of your session tomorrow?" Respond. (Week 13: Saying No and Saving Face)

> The occupational therapy supervisor says to you, the therapist: "You know, your treatment goals are all Greek to me!" Respond. (Week 11: Supervision: Taking It)

Often during one or another of the class hours, didactic material from various theorists serves as an organizing focus for discussion, reflection, and practice. Some of these theorists are Adler (1931), Brammer (1973), Buber (1965), Cash (1983), Egan (1986), Fisher and Brown (1988), Gladstein (1987), Goldstein and Michaels (1985), Kagan (1983), Katz (1963), Knapp (1972), Muldary (1983), Pfeiffer and Jones (1974), Reik (1949), Rogers (1957, 1958) and Tubesing and Tubesing (1973). Several cartoons from the works of Larson (1984) and Callahan (1989) also provide provocative material for commentary about interpersonal gaffes and foibles.

Because reflection and practice are so fundamental to learning to communicate, students are expected to complete entries in personal journals on a regular basis. The journal assignments include the following: (a) complete a self-assessment of your interactional style, (b) respond to the results of the self-assessment, (c) write about an experience with active listening, (d) write about your personal "hot buttons" (interpersonal situations that you anticipate will be especially difficult for you). Write the worst possible scenario that you can imagine, and then describe how you might better deal with the same situation, (e) write about an experience with limit setting, (f) write about an experience in which you used negative inquiry.

Discussion

One student's comments served as a catalyst for developing this course. Comments from a number of students who took the course support offering it again.

> Sure, I had some idea that being caring and understanding might enhance my life as a person and a professional, but I was not quite sure how to do it. Through stories and role play, I learned to give an understanding response and empathize with others. I reflected about my own feelings and thought so I tuned in to myself as well as to the feelings of others. I learned the meaning of respect, caring, and trust. As a result of this course, I feel that I will be better able to respond in the clinic and in my life.

> As occupational therapy students, we learn a lot from textbooks. This learning is important. We do not, however, explore the most important tool: the therapeutic use of self. There is no textbook that tells how to act toward a particular patient, what one should say or do. To understand why a person acts or feels in a particular way, memorizing from a textbook is not helpful. Sharing stories and experiences is a better way to think about and explore the worlds of others. In interpersonal skills, the environment was one in which we felt OK about exploring and making mistakes.

> Being a good health care provider goes beyond the technical aspects of health care. Discussing abstract concepts related to interpersonal skills does not give a real sense of what it is like to respect, care for, and trust someone. Stories portray interpersonal encounters in a way that makes abstract concepts real.

It was an awakening to see the manner in which students struggled with the role play sessions during the first few weeks of the course. Although most students could clearly articulate a concept or strategy about which they needed to be mindful, many found it difficult to put these concepts into practice. As the course progressed, however, so did they. The success of the course in the first year has led to the decision to offer it again, twice during the fall semester, as both a junior and senior elective. ▲

Acknowledgment

We thank Donald A. Davison, MA, OTR, Chair of the Occupational Therapy Department, for his encouragement and support.

References

Adler, A. (1931). *What life should mean to you.* Boston: Little, Brown.

Brammer, L. M. (1973). *The helping relationship.* Englewood Cliffs, NJ: Prentice-Hall.

Buber, M. (1965). *Between man and man.* New York: Macmillan.

Callahan, R. (1989). *Don't worry he won't get far on foot.* New York: Vintage.

Cash, R. W. (1983). The Human Resources Development Model. In D. Larson (Ed.), *Teaching psychological skills: Models for giving psychology away* (pp. 246–270). Monterey: Brooks/Cole.

Egan, G. (1986). *The skilled helper: A systematic approach to effective helping.* Monterey: Brooks/Cole.

Fisher, R., & Brown, S. (1988). *Getting together: Building relationships as we negotiate.* New York: Penguin.

Gladstein, G. A. (1987). *Empathy and counseling: Explorations in theory and research.* New York: Springer-Verlag.

Goldstein, A. P., & Michaels, G. Y. (1985). *Empathy: Development, training, and consequences.* New Jersey: Erlbaum.

Kagan, N. (1983). Interpersonal process recall: Basic methods and recent research. In D. Larson (Ed.), *Teaching psychological skills: Models for giving psychology away* (pp. 229–246). Monterey: Brooks/Cole.

Katz, R. (1963) *Empathy: Its nature and uses.* London: Free Press of Glencoe.

Knapp, M. L. (1972). *Nonverbal communication in human interaction.* New York: Holt, Rinehart, & Winston.

Larson, G (1984). *The far side gallery.* New York: Andrews, McMeel, Parker.

Maclay, E. (1977). *Green winter: Celebrations of old age.* New York: Reader's Digest Press.

Mosey, A. C. (1981). *Occupational therapy: Configuration of a profession.* New York: Raven.

Muldary, T. (1983). *Interpersonal relations for health professionals: A social skills approach.* New York: Macmillan.

Peloquin, S. M. (1989). Sustaining the art of practice in occupational therapy. *American Journal of Occupational Therapy, 43,* 219–226.

Peloquin, S. M. (1990). The patient–therapist relationship in occupational therapy: Understanding visions and images. *American Journal of Occupational Therapy, 44,* 3–21.

Pfeiffer, J. W., & Jones, J. J. (1974). *A handbook of structured experiences for human relations training.* LaJolla, California: University Associates.

Plum, A. (1981). Communication as skill: A critique and alternative proposal. *Journal of Humanistic Psychology, 21,* 3–19.

Reik, T. (1949). *Listening with the third ear.* New York: Farrar, Strauss.

Rogers, C. (1957). The necessary and sufficient conditions of therapeutic personality change. *Journal of Consulting Psychology, 21,* 95–103.

Rogers, C. (1958). The characteristics of a helping relationship. *Personnel and Guidance Journal, 37,* 6–16.

Tubesing, D. A. & Tubesing, N. L. (1973). *Tune In—Empathy training workshop.* Duluth, Minnesota: Listening Group.

Suggested Readings

Beers, C. (1917). *A mind that found itself.* New York: Longmans, Green.

Beisser, A. (1989). *Flying without wings: Personal reflections on becoming disabled.* New York: Doubleday.

Belknap, M. M., Blau, R. A., & Grossman, R. N. (1975). *Case studies and methods in humanistic medical care: Some preliminary findings.* San Francisco: Institute for the Study of Humanistic Medicine.

Benzinger, B. F. (1969). *The prison of my mind.* New York: Walker and Company.

Brice, J. (1978). Empathy lost. *Harvard Medical Journal, 60,* 28–32.

Browne, K., & Freeling, P. (1976). *The doctor–patient relationship.* New York: Churchill Livingstone.

Carlova, J., & Ruggles, O. (1946). *The healing heart.* New York: Messner.

Casell, E. (1988). *Talking with patients, Volume 1: The theory of doctor–patient communication.* Cambridge: MIT Press.

Coles, R. (1989). *The call of stories.* Boston: Houghton Mifflin.

Engel, G. (1976). Too little science. The paradox of modern medicine's crisis. *Pharos, 39,* 127–131.

Fay, E. V., & March, I. (1947). Occupational therapy in general and special hospitals. In H. S. Willard & C. S. Spackman (Eds.), *Principles of occupational therapy* (pp. 118–137). Philadelphia: Lippincott.

Flagg, P. (1923). *The patient's viewpoint.* Milwaukee: Bruce Publishing.

Gebolys, E. (1990). Inadequacies, inequities, and inanities in modern medicine—A personal experience. *Occupational Therapy Forum, 12,* 6–7, 13–18.

Harris, B., & Stripling, S. (1980) The patient on the receiving end, out of control. *Cancer Bulletin, 32,* 20–21.

Heller, J., & Speed, V. (1986). *No laughing matter.* New York: Avon.

Hodgins, E. (1964). Whatever became of the healing art? *Annals of the New York Academy of Sciences, 164,* 838–846.

Jacques, F. (1983).*Verdict pending: A patient representative's intervention.* Capistrano, California: Capistrano Press.

Jourard, S. (1964). *The transparent self: Self disclosure and well being.* New York: Van Nostrand Reinhold.

Kafka, F. (1986). *The metamorphosis* (S. Corngold, Trans. and Ed.). New York: Bantam.

Kleinman, A. (1988). *The illness narratives: Suffering, healing, and the human condition.* New York: Basic.

Lear, H. (1980). *Heartsounds.* New York: Simon & Schuster.

Leder, D. (1984). Medicine and paradigms of embodiment. *Journal of Medicine and Philosophy, 9,* 29–43.

Lee, L. (1987). Transcendence. In M. Saxton & F. Howe (Eds.), *With wings: An anthology of literature by and about women with disabilities.* New York: The Feminist Press.

Leete, E. (1987). The treatment of schizophrenia: A patient's perspective. *Hospital and Community Psychiatry, 38,* 486–491.

L. E. P. (July, 1987). *Reader's Digest* 53.

Longcope, W. (1962). Methods and medicine. In W. H. Davenport (Ed.), *The good physician: A treasure of medicine.* New York: Macmillan.

Mizrahi, T. (1986). *Getting rid of patients: Contradictions in the socialization of physicians.* New Brunswick: Rutgers University Press.

Moore, A. (1978). *The missing text: Humane patient care.* Australia: Melbourne University Press.

Murphy, R. F.(1987). *The body silent.* New York: Henry Holt.

Nicky, (1982). A visit to a renovated clinic. *Journal of the American Medical Association, 247,* 1906.

Peabody, B. (1986). *The screaming room: A mother's journal of her son's struggle with AIDS—A true story of love, dedication, and courage.* New York: Avon.

Peabody, F. W. (1930). *Doctor and patient papers on the relationship of the physician to men and institutions.* New York: Macmillan.

Pekkanen, J. (1988). *MD: Doctors talk about themselves.* New York: Del Publishing.

Pellegrino, E. (1979). *Humanism and the physician.* Knoxville: University of Tennessee Press.

Peters, T., & Austin, N. (1985). *A passion for excellence: The leadership difference.* New York: Random House.

Remen, N. (1975). *The masculine principle, the feminine principle and humanistic medicine.* San Francisco: The Institute for Study of Humanistic Medicine.

Rogers, C. R. (1957). The necessary and sufficient conditions of therapeutic personality change. *Journal of Consulting Psychology, 21,* 95–103.

Sacks, O. (1983). *Awakenings.* New York: E. P. Dutton.

Sacks, O. (1984). *A leg to stand on.* New York: Harper & Row.

Sarason, S. B. (1985). *Caring and compassion in clinical practice.* San Francisco: Jossey-Bass.

Sarton, M. (1988). *After the stroke: A journal.* New York: Norton.

Saxton, M. (1987). Seeking help and love. In M. Saxton & F. Howe (Eds.), *With wings: An anthology of literature by and about women with disabilities.* New York: The Feminist Press.

Slaby, A. A., & Glickman, A. S. (1986). Adaptation of physicians to managing life-threatening illness. *Integrative Psychiatry, 4,* 162–165.

Thomas, L. (1983). The Tucson zoo. In *The medusa and the snail: Notes of a biology watcher.* New York: Viking Press.

Thomas, L. (1983). *The youngest science: Notes of a medicine-watcher.* New York: Viking Press.

Trillin, A. S. (1981). Of dragons and garden peas: A cancer patient talks to doctors. *New England Journal of Medicine, 304,* 699–701.

Triplett, J. L. (1969). Empathy is. *Nursing Clinics of North America, 4,* 673–681.

Williams, W. C. (1948). *The autobiography of William Carlos Williams.* New York: Random House.

The Issue Is

Communication Skills: Why Not Turn to a Skills Training Model?

Suzanne M. Peloquin

Suzanne M. Peloquin, PhD, OTR, is Associate Professor, Department of Occupational Therapy, School of Allied Health Sciences, University of Texas Medical Branch at Galveston, 301 University Boulevard, Galveston, Texas 77555-1028.

This article was accepted for publication November 28, 1994.

The standards for professional education found in the *Essentials and Guidelines for an Accredited Educational Program for the Occupational Therapist* (American Occupational Therapy Association [AOTA], 1991) constitute an outline of the substantive learning that practitioners consider important (the essentials) as well as suggested methods for fostering that learning (the guidelines). One of the essentials is that a program prepare the occupational therapist to "incorporate values and attitudes congruent with the profession's standards and ethics." (AOTA, 1991, p. 4) Although these values and attitudes are not specified in the *Essentials*, they are the subject of another official document, *Core Values and Attitudes of Occupational Therapy Practice* (AOTA, 1993), and they cluster around seven concepts: altruism, equality, freedom, justice, dignity, truth, and prudence. According to the combined wisdom of the two documents, students must learn to express and implement these fundamental values, and educators must facilitate that learning. This mandate grows more pressing at a time when the health care delivery system challenges these core values.

Educators who refer to the *Essentials* in order to meet the mandate soon see the broad range of educational tools at their disposal and foster "appropriate learning experiences and curriculum sequencing to develop the competencies" of students (AOTA, 1991, p. 5). The *Essentials* also elaborates on program content. Three program requirements correspond with the development of attitudes and values: liberal arts content that will facilitate communication skills; the use of self, dyadic, and group interaction; and the understanding of professional ethics. Noting the first content area—communication skills—educators may turn to the behavioral sciences for textbooks or handbooks that derive

from well-established training programs. The choice seems logical, the approach appropriate. Most educators will not consider why the *Essentials* fails to mention the behavioral sciences as a suitable resource.

The question that drives this discussion is simple: Why not draw from the behavioral sciences to teach communication skills to occupational therapy students? A critical look at educational strategies known under the general category of communication skills training offers a straightforward answer. The skills training model, in its focus on performance, holds little promise for developing attitudes and values in students. Any model that shapes a way of doing may fall short when the desired outcome is a way of being.

One core value—dignity—can serve as illustration and focal point for this discussion. A therapist who values human dignity is said to express it as "an attitude of empathy and respect for self and others" (AOTA, 1993, p. 1086). Communication skills training often builds on the assumption that one will learn empathy in the process of mastering skills in communication. That assumption invites reflection. The issue is that communication skills training is not

apt to help students develop empathy, and it seems important that educators consider the limitations of such training.

Skills Training: At High Risk for Reductionism

Walters (1990) coined a term in education when she claimed that teachers "vulcanize" (p. 448) their students. She said that "any fan of the old 'Star Trek' television series knows there is something remarkably gripping about the character Spock" (p. 448) from the fictional planet Vulcan. Spock had laser-sharp logical skills but lacked feeling and imagination. Walters argued that many educators teach students to be proficient in Vulcan-like thinking. The problem, she said, is that good thinkers are not Vulcan-like; they also use imagination and insight. There is a strong resonance between Walters' discussion of vulcanization and Schön's (1983) characterization of the model of technical rationality that denies the artistry of professional practice. The trend toward logical analysis and technical competence pervades the behavioral sciences as well. Whether one calls this reduction *vulcanizing* or *rationalizing*, the education of values shrivels within communication skills training.

When Rogers (1972) discussed empathy as a necessary condition for practice, he hoped to lead practitioners to this deeply personal action:

> It means entering the private world of the other and becoming thoroughly at home in it. It involves being sensitive, moment to moment, to the changing felt meanings which flow in this other person, to the fear or rage or tenderness or confusion or whatever, that he/she is experiencing. It means temporarily living in his/her life, moving about in it delicately without making judgments. (p. 3)

Rogers (1965) regretted the many distortions of empathy that he saw: "It seems to me that most of our professional training programmes make it *more* difficult for the individual to be himself, and more likely that he will play a professional role" (p. 106). The argument seems valid.

Students eager to learn how to empathize often learn instead about *communication skills*. A typical format for such learning resembles the module designed by Brammer (1973):

- Skill cluster 1: Listening skills
- Skill cluster 2: Leading
- Skill cluster 3: Reflecting
- Skill cluster 4: Summarizing
- Skill cluster 5: Confronting
- Skill cluster 6: Interpreting
- Skill cluster 7: Informing

Brammer (1973) introduced his microskills training approach as "analogous to skills training in a sport such as golf, in which one learns the fundamental skills of stance, grip, and swing" (p. 68). Brammer's list gives one pause even if it includes many actions with which a practitioner must be skilled: It fails to mention the fundamental act of understanding another person. Brammer admitted only that the problem that follows breaking down an action is one of putting its parts together into a smooth and natural performance.

Plum (1981) disagreed. He thought the problems with skill training insurmountable: "Skill approaches to communication training mistakenly place skillfulness, rather than meaning, at the heart of personal communication" (p. 3). Much to Gladstein's (1987) dismay, practitioners have sought to prove the efficacy of communication skills training with methods that split the gestures from the heart of empathy: "Research concerning empathy has . . . created measures that have tended to isolate the affective from the cognitive components" (p. 5).

Training for Empathic Responses

A sampling of training strategies may illustrate the inadequacy of this rationalized view of empathy. The Human Resources Development program (Carkhuff, 1972) is, according to Cash (1983), the most widely used in professional and paraprofessional training. Human resources trainees learn to analyze interpersonal situations and pro-

duce responses designed to convey increasing levels of empathy. A level-one response, for example, is one in which "the verbal and behavioral expressions of the helper either do not attend to or detract significantly from the verbal and behavioral expressions of the helpee" (Goldstein & Michaels, 1985, p. 199). In a more empathic level-three response, "the expressions of the helper in response to the expressions of the helpee are essentially interchangeable with those of the helpee in that they express essentially the same affect and meaning" (Goldstein & Michaels, p. 199). Responding at level three, a trainee would identify the feeling and the problem of a person and then accurately reflect both, with any natural-sounding variation of the "You feel _____ because _____" construction.

Training that produces more attentive responses to others seems promising. Instructed to move past either inaccurate or cold responses, trainees in human resources development differentiate their communications and then practice during role play (Cash, 1983). A successful trainee consistently responds at level three or higher by the end of training. However, Lambert and DeJulio (1977) summarized their careful critique of the extensive outcome research done on human resources development training programs and stated: "It is difficult to keep your eye on the donut because of the size of the hole" (p. 86). They argued that the gains made in training did not generalize to more practical situations.

Often, students hope to learn empathic responses that will enhance pragmatic functions, such as the patient interview. Typically, students learn snippets of the Human Relations Development model (Carkhuff, 1972) along with portions of another model, the Interpersonal Process Recall (IPR) for which Kagan (1983) described his initial aim:

> The core of the IPR process is reviewing a videotape or audiotape in order to recall one's thoughts, feelings, goals, aspirations, bodily sensations, and a host of other covert processes and describing these processes as explicitly as possible during the tape reviews. (p. 229)

But the IPR model is typically used more narrowly: to identify and yield effective interviews rather than to stimu-

late reflection.

The following patient account suggests that even with a pragmatic function like the interview in mind, the problem of putting the parts together in a meaningful way can be vexing:

> Running late to class, I hit a pavement hole and fell. So badly battered and bloodied was my knee that I dragged myself into the emergency clinic of a nearby hospital. . . . After about twenty minutes I was called into an inner office by a rosy-faced young man whose stethoscope in the pocket of his white coat established his identity and professional authority.
> "So!" he said pleasantly, scanning not my face but my face sheet. "You are _____" (my name).
> "Yes," I said.
> "Hm," he said. "You are _____" (my age).
> "Yes," said I.
> "Do you have children?" he asked.
> "Yes," said I. "One."
> "Good!" he said approvingly. "Is he married?"
> "Um hum," said I.
> "Do you have any grandchildren?" he asked. This was followed by several other socially innocuous and totally irrelevant (to me and my throbbing knee) questions.
> Suddenly I caught on. In this good teaching hospital this aspiring doctor had probably recently had a lecture either to the effect that a doctor should "relate to the person and not just to the disease" or that "first you establish a relationship with your patient." . . . But it had not been made clear to him that, when the person comes suffering with the disease, it must be this combination of the problem and its personal hurt that must be the simultaneous, interwoven focus of any caring inquiry (Perlman, 1979, pp. 141–142).

When practitioners use skill components to make superficial connections, they substitute social chitchat for empathy.

Training for Affective Sensitivity

Most persons will acknowledge that a person who follows the lines of any protocol will skim the surface of empathy. Most know that they must show some appreciation of the feeling of another if they are to be seen as understanding. This appreciation is known as *affective sensitivity* (Kagan, 1983). Most training for affective sensitivity emphasizes those nonverbal behaviors that convey emotions; such training also teaches the cognitive aspects of the construct. Highly technical terms such as *affect displays, kinesics, proxemics, paralan-*

guage, *illustrators, adaptors, regulators,* and *vocalizations* organize the literature on nonverbal communication while breaking it down into learnable parts and clusters (Knapp, 1972).

When practitioners *train* to use the complex nonverbal clusters that express feelings, they ready themselves narrowly. They may recall the words of Egan (1977) who suggested that helpers use the mnemonic SOLER when approaching their patients:

- S: Face the other person *squarely*. This is the basic posture of involvement.
- O: Adopt an *open* posture.
- L: *Lean* toward the other. This is another sign of presence.
- E: Maintain good *eye contact*.
- R: Try to be at home or relatively *relaxed* while attending. (p. 115)

One apprehends in SOLER a preference for a formula rather than a cultivation of sensitivity. Rational cues then replace a more empathic way of being there.

Hoping to nudge helpers closer to seeing the inadequacy of any skills training orientation, whether verbal or nonverbal, Plum (1981) cited R. D. Laing (1969):

> It is not so easy for one person to give another a cup of tea. If a lady gives me a cup of tea, she might be showing off her teapot, or her tea-set; she might be trying to put me in a good mood in order to get something out of me; she may be trying to get me to like her; she may be wanting me as an ally for her own purposes against others. She might pour tea from a pot into a cup and shove out her hand with cup and saucer in it, whereupon I am expected to grab them within two seconds before they will become dead weight. The action could be a mechanical one in which there is no recognition of me in it. A cup of tea could be handed *me* without me being *given a cup of tea.* (p. 106)

When would-be helpers hand their patients words and gestures while not trying to understand, the approach feels mechanical. The question that patients then ask is not whether practitioners mean to harm, but whether they want to care.

Conclusion

Sarason (1985) saw the consequence of technical approaches: "What disturbs people, what makes the wall around them seem so impermeable, is their sense that helping actions are powered by the language of social ritual and not by any real grappling with the process of understanding" (p. 188). A patient's wall building seems more than justified in light of these outrageous suggestions from Korneluk (1985):

> There are some ideas that you can incorporate into your personal style to improve your patients' perception of you and lead them to think of your practice as being totally competent. . . . By using his or her name and referring to the chart from memory you appear more competent and project a warm, personal touch to your encounter. People like having their names spoken; it establishes a positive relationship right from the beginning. . . . Patients appreciate eye contact, and it projects the feeling that you are very attentive. . . . Remember, you are the star, since patients are coming to see you. (pp. 225–228)

Katz (1963) judged health care practitioners who underidentify with their patients to be "rationalistic empathizers" (p. 164) and contended that many say the words and make the gestures of empathic communication, but that the personal element of the encounter is lost. The picture of one so trained is that of a person without feelings and sensitivity; it is the picture of a "Vulcan."

Rogers (1965) described the enactment of empathy in a way that bared its essence. He described it as a way of entering into the inner worlds of other persons. If occupational therapy practitioners are to empathize with others, they must engage in forms of learning that lead them to value the personal dignity that invites such encounters. A skills training model may offer much that is valuable, but it cannot promise to develop the fundamental value that expresses itself as empathy. Perhaps the message of the *Essentials* is: Students are more apt to learn values from approaches that inspire a way of being. ▲

References

American Occupational Therapy Association. (1991). *Essentials and guidelines for an accredited educational program for the occupational therapist.* Rockville, MD: American Occupational Therapy Association.

American Occupational Therapy Association. (1993). Core values and attitudes of occupational therapy practice. *American Journal of Occupational Therapy, 47,* 1085–1086.

Brammer, L. M. (1973). *The helping relationship.* Englewood Cliffs, NJ: Prentice-Hall.

Carkhuff, R. R. (1972). The development of systematic human resource development models. *Counseling Psychologist, 3,* 4–10.

Cash, R. W. (1983). The human resources development model. In D. Larson (Ed.), *Teaching psychological skills: Models for giving psychology away* (pp. 245–270). Monterey, CA: Brooks/Cole.

Egan, G. (1977). *You & me: The skills of communicating and relating to others.* Belmont, CA: Wadsworth.

Gladstein, G. A. (1987). *Empathy and counseling: Exploration in theory and research.* New York: Springer-Verlag.

Goldstein, A. P., & Michaels, G. Y. (1985). *Empathy: Development, training, and consequences.* New York: Macmillan.

Kagan, N. (1983). Interpersonal process recall: Basic methods and recent research. In Dale Larson (Ed.), Teaching psychological skills: *Models for giving psychology away* (pp. 229–245). Monterey, CA: Brooks/Cole.

Katz, R. L. (1963). *Empathy: Its nature and uses.* London: Free Press of Glencoe.

Knapp, M. L. (1972). *Nonverbal communication in human interaction.* New York: Holt, Rinehart, & Winston.

Korneluk, G. N. (1985). *Practice enhancement: The physician's guide to success in private practice.* New York: Macmillan.

Laing, R. D. (1969). *Self and others.* London: Penguin.

Lambert, M. J., & DeJulio, S. S. (1977). Outcome research in Carkhuff's human resource development training programs: Where is the donut? *Counseling Psychologist, 6,* 79–86.

Perlman, H. H. (1979). *Relationship: The heart of helping people.* Chicago: University of Chicago Press.

Plum, A. (1981). Communication as skill: A critique and alternative proposal. *Journal of Humanistic Psychology, 21*(4), 3–19.

Rogers, C. R. (1965). The therapeutic relationship: Recent theory and research. *Australian Journal of Psychology, 17,* 95–108.

Rogers, C. R. (1972). Bringing together ideas and feelings. *Learning Today, 5*(2), 32–43.

Sarason, S. (1985). *Caring and compassion in clinical practice.* San Francisco: Jossey-Bass.

Schön, D. A. (1983). The reflective practitioner: *How professionals think in action.* New York: Basic.

Walters, K. (1990). Critical thinking, rationality, and the vulcanization of students. *Journal of Higher Education, 61,* 448–467.

THE ISSUE IS provides a forum for debate and discussion of occupational therapy issues and related topics. The Contributing Editor of this section, Julia Van Deusen, strives to have both sides of an issue addressed. Readers are encouraged to submit manuscripts discussing opposite points of view or new topics. All manuscripts are subject to peer review. Submit three copies to Elaine Viseltear, Editor.

Published articles reflect the opinion of the authors and are selected on the basis of interest to the profession and quality of the discussion.

The Patient–Therapist Relationship in Occupational Therapy: Understanding Visions and Images

Suzanne M. Peloquin

Key Words: literature • professional competence • professional–patient relations

The patient–therapist relationship in occupational therapy has been a blend of competence and caring with the emphasis fluctuating over the years between these two features. When patients tell stories about their experiences, they reveal widely differing views of occupational therapists, partly because of the different ways therapists manifest competence and caring during patient–therapist interactions. Images from stories suggest that some therapists unwittingly disappoint their patients. This paper examines the patient–therapist relationship as envisioned by therapists and patients to help occupational therapists recommit to the patient as a vital partner in a collaborative relationship.

Suzanne M. Peloquin, MA, OTR, is an Assistant Professor at the School of Allied Health Sciences, The University of Texas Medical Branch, Galveston, Texas, 77551.

This article was accepted for publication March 7, 1989.

The stories patients tell about their experiences with occupational therapists often tell more about their views than structured responses to surveys. The following fictional story tells much about one patient–therapist relationship:

> Brunhilde, the misplaced Viking Lady, comes tapping on my door every afternoon in an effort to intimidate me into going to Occupational Therapy. She marches around the seventh floor telling all the patients that their doctor has "ordered" Occupational Therapy and they must come IMMEDIATELY. She herds them out in the hall and they mill around until she lines them up in two columns and goosesteps them out the door. (Rebeta-Burditt, 1977, p. 114)

A fuller reading of the story reveals that this patient, Cassie, accurately perceives expressions of concern from other health care professionals. Her satirical barbs target those whose demands for control and order threaten her autonomy. Because Brunhilde seems uncaring, the image of the occupational therapist in this story is disturbing.

Clinically, patients derive images of their therapists from their interactions with them. Image forming as a process includes an exchange: The therapist brings to each exchange some understanding, or vision, of what a therapeutic relationship (and perhaps what a "good patient") should be, and the patient brings needs, memories of past experiences, and expectations of how a helpful caregiver should behave. The exchange of needs, visions, and expectations helps to shape the image that each person will hold of the other. In the above story, Cassie is frustrated by an occupational therapist who does not demonstrate the kind of personal concern that she wants and expects. She sees a paternalistic therapist, an intimidating Viking Lady. The novel does not reveal the vision of the therapeutic relationship that the therapist brought to this exchange. One can only wonder what happened beyond the patient's unmet expectations to yield such a negative image.

The therapeutic relationship promoted in occupational therapy has been an evolving blend of competence and caring. Therapists have interacted with patients in a variety of ways, depending in part on their interpretation of the occupational therapy vision. It follows that images of occupational therapists in patients' stories have also varied. This paper will examine the patient–therapist relationship envisioned by therapists and experienced by patients. Thoughtful consideration of both views—the visions therapists have of the relationship and the images patients hold of their therapists—can remind practitioners that concern about the patient as a person remains essential to effective practice.

The Patient–Therapist Relationship: In Search of the Occupational Therapy Vision

Perhaps no source better illustrates the evolution of the profession's understanding of the patient–therapist relationship than *Willard and Spackman's Occupational Therapy*. From the first edition (Willard & Spackman, 1947) to the sixth edition (Hopkins & Smith, 1983), this text has presented contributions from therapists working in a variety of practice arenas. *Willard and Spackman* has been a primary tool in the education of occupational therapy students and has often served as a therapist's first introduction to the vision of the therapeutic relationship.

The therapeutic relationship, however, has been treated in a fragmented way in this basic text. Between 1947 and 1983, no chapter has specifically addressed the therapeutic relationship. No references are made in either the table of contents or the index to concepts such as *rapport* or *relationship* or to key relational words such as *empathy* or *trust*. The 1947 edition has brief sections entitled "Approach to the Patient," "Personality Qualifications," "Normal Atmosphere," and "The Attitude of the Therapist." The 1983 edition has pertinent sections called "The Therapist," "Observation," "Humanistic Approaches," and "Psychological Considerations." A discussion of patient–therapist communication as it affects the evaluation process is listed in the index under the heading Communication, and a discrete section entitled "Therapeutic Relationship" is in the chapter on functional restoration. It seems significant, however, that within a definitive text on occupational therapy, one can find the profession's vision of the therapeutic relationship only after a chapter-by-chapter search.

If each treatment chapter addressed relational considerations for the patient population in question, one could argue that the concept of the therapeutic relationship is so basic that it permeates the text. But this is clearly not the case. Most of the material articulates the assumptions, theories, and methodologies essential to the application of occupation. Although this emphasis is essential in an occupational therapy text, the minimal acknowledgment that occupational therapy occurs within the context of the patient–therapist relationship suggests the curiously marginal status of this fact. Because fragments of information about the therapeutic relationship are scattered throughout several chapters, the reader cannot gain a clear understanding of the vision from this one source. The fragmented manner in which the patient–therapist relationship is covered compromises its significance and clarity.

The Evolving Vision: From Competence to Care

The vision articulated in *Willard and Spackman's Occupational Therapy* has changed over the years, largely through changes in emphasis. Earlier contributors advocated skill-oriented and professional (impersonal) patient–therapist relationships; the emphasis was on competence. Later contributors focused on the essentially personal character of the patient–therapist relationship, with the emphasis on care.

For example, in the 1947 edition of *Willard and Spackman*, Wade characterized the development of the therapeutic relationship in treating the mentally ill in a rather impersonal way:

> The development of a good psychiatric approach does not occur spontaneously, nor is it a natural gift but, like many other accomplishments, it is acquired through diligent effort, study and experience. (p. 83)

Wade viewed a good patient–therapist relationship as an achievement attained by a skilled therapist who could "command respect, admiration, hope and confidence" (p. 83). She identified "courage, patience, tolerance and friendliness" as innate personal characteristics that could be directed toward the achievement of a good approach (p. 83). Wade additionally characterized the successful therapist as one who had mastered two specific skills that supported patient equilibrium. First was the ability to make a "tactful approach," one in which "adjustment is always made to the patient by the worker" (p. 84). Wade explained the rationale for this guarded approach: "These patients are hypersensitive to implications expressed in words, by tone of voice, mannerism or facial expression" (p. 84). Second, the therapist needed "complete self-control in order to prevent untimely expression of a spontaneous emotional reaction" (p. 84). Self-control and personal adjustment seemed critical to patient equilibrium; spontaneity and personal expression were suspect.

Other skills entailed reaching out to the patient, but always within the context of professional objectivity. The therapist had to identify with the patient, but at the same time maintain an objective attitude: "The technic [sic] of doing this is similar to that used by the adult in correlating his thoughts with those of a child" (Wade, 1947, p. 84). The therapeutic goal was primary; caring expressions were a means to that end. The therapist needed to be a good listener, for example, because "it is frequently necessary to play this role" (Wade, 1947, p. 84). The patient–therapist relationship was to be kept "within normal limits" and "restricted to matters of impersonal interest" (Wade, 1947, p. 85). The bottom line during interactions with the mentally ill was that one remain "impersonal in relationships" (Wade, 1947, p. 84).

This emphasis on competence was not restricted to practice in mental health. Fay and March (1947) discussed the development of the therapeutic relationship in both general and special hospitals:

> Skill in making the professional approach to each patient for occupational therapy may come more easily to some than to others, but it comes with experience in correlating the patient's history with the character as revealed by his face to one who is interested in enlisting the patient's co-operation. (pp. 124–125)

The relationship had to be professional. Toward that end, Fay and March enumerated several guidelines for a suitable approach. The following guidelines are representative of the list's precision and direction:

Do's

3. Stand or sit where you can be seen easily.
4. Be encouraging and hopeful and foster a desire in the patient to get well.
5. Be understandingly sympathetic.
6. Be friendly and sincere.
7. Be courteous, not flippant or bold.
11. Be patient and resourceful.
12. Be impersonally personal.

Don't's

3. Don't show alarm, horror or sorrow.
5. Don't be physically objectionable by body odor, the use of strong perfume or by having the clothes permeated with cigarette smoke.
7. Don't argue. Be a good listener.
8. Don't talk of depressing or distressing subjects.
9. Don't make promises that cannot be kept.
10. Don't hit or jar the bed.
12. Don't show racial, religious or political prejudices. (pp. 125–126)

The predominant vision of the patient–therapist relationship in this 1947 edition reflected a self-conscious striving for precise skills that could professionalize the patient–therapist relationship. Personal, warm traits were seen as tools requiring guidance, monitoring, and objectification. Perhaps the closest any contributor in the 1947 edition came to the idea of personal investment and care in relationships with patients was Gleave in her chapter on pediatric services:

> The occupational therapist should be an understanding, friendly and cheerful person. . . . Ability to talk *with* children rather than *to* or *at* them is an asset. Every effort should be made to bring out the child's ideas, to get him to express himself freely and naturally. In all contacts with the patient, the therapist should strive to keep the tone of her voice pleasant and well modulated. She must make the child feel that she is his friend while holding his respect and maintaining discipline when problems arise. (p. 148)

Gleave alone alluded to the concept of friendship in the therapeutic relationship. Her emphasis on a caring expression seemed acceptable in 1947 within the context of working with children, for whom, perhaps,

the need to project a professional image seemed less crucial.

By the 1983 edition of *Willard and Spackman's Occupational Therapy,* however, the term *therapeutic relationship* had taken root, and the therapist's caring attitude had assumed greater significance than personality traits or interactional skills. As if in recognition of prior emphasis on competence and professionalism, Hopkins and Tiffany (1983) cited a new image: Purtilo's characterization of "the personal–professional self" (p. 95). Purtilo (1978), a physical therapist, proposed a synthesis of personal and professional characteristics to facilitate the therapeutic relationship. She tried to minimize conflicts for therapists struggling with personal–professional tension in relationships with patients. This brief portion of Purtilo's (1978) characterization reveals her vision:

> [The personal–professional self] incorporates actions that communicate caring into the patient health professional interactions; he recognizes efficiency as a trait which can express caring when it does not impose rigid limits on the interaction.
>
> He is interested in the patient as a person with values, needs, and beliefs, but does not encourage a relationship that will lead to over-dependence (detrimental dependence). (p. 148)

This more balanced view of the therapeutic relationship communicated a sense of helping. Hopkins and Tiffany (1983) believed that patients need to feel that they can be helped and argued that "the therapist in a treatment setting is, by definition, a helper" (p. 94). The helping process required personal trust—a trust built on confidence in and respect for the patient:

> Without the establishment of trust between the client and therapist, it is unlikely that a truly collaborative effort will be possible. . . . The therapist's own self-confidence, the therapist's ability to be honest and open in the relationship, and the extent to which the therapist is able to communicate "unconditional positive regard" and empathy for the client will affect the client's ability to invest trust in the relationship. (pp. 94–95)

Tiffany (1983) underscored her view of the therapist's role: "Occupational therapy is attuned to the principle of facilitating the client's own personal search for purpose, meaning, and self-actualization" (p. 291). Open communication between the therapist and patient seemed critical to understanding the patient's purpose and personal values. Smith and Tiffany (1983) elaborated: "The communication process . . . lays a foundation for rapport and trust. The client needs to feel that communications have been heard and understood by someone who has not only some empathy but also some knowledge and skill" (pp. 144–145). A personal relationship was critical to this new vision. It was the *relationship* that might well "determine the success or failure of the treatment plan" (Hopkins & Tiffany, 1983, p. 94), and within that relationship, "activities are used as facilitators for transactions between people" (Hopkins & Tiffany, p. 95). This singular distinction ought never be forgotten; occupational therapy's vision of "being with" is essentially a vision of "doing with."

This later vision of the therapeutic relationship, with its emphasis on care, on the importance of each person, and on helping, transcended the awkward and self-conscious vision of earlier years. Both visions grounded themselves in competence and caring, and both highlighted competencies and styles of caring thought (in their respective eras) to be important and effective. A young profession, striving to be recognized as scientific, might emphasize competence. A more secure profession, leery of the objectification inherent in scientific practice, might more readily emphasize care.

When one pieces together the ideas of 1947 and 1983 regarding the therapeutic relationship, the ensuing vision lends itself to much individual interpretation. One therapist may feel that earlier directives to be "impersonally personal" should yield to more recent appeals for warmth; another may favor a relationship marked by more traditional objectivity and distance. If therapists demonstrate competence and caring in different ways in contemporary practice, this is consistent with their having been exposed to a fragmented and evolving vision of the patient–therapist relationship over the years.

From Therapist's Vision to Patient's Image

Stories about occupational therapists tell much about their relationships with patients. In this next section, I will attempt to explore stories from the 1940s through the 1980s that develop the therapeutic relationship, citing the stories wherever possible. Although in a previous article (Peloquin, 1989) I emphasized that fiction can contribute powerfully to therapists' understanding of their functions, I here draw primarily from nonfiction so that the stories will ring truer to those who might dismiss fictional accounts as fantasy.

A Pioneer: Ora Ruggles

One biography in particular presents a therapist with a clear vision of what she believes the therapeutic relationship should be. *The Healing Heart* (Carlova & Ruggles, 1946) portrays a competent and caring reconstruction aide and pioneer, Ora Ruggles. Ruggles's bold and humane vision contrasts markedly with that of her 1940s contemporaries; it reflects a patient–therapist relationship more characteristic of the vision of the 1980s. Her drive to relate to patients

is clear: "It is not enough to give a patient something to do with his hands. You must reach for the heart as well as the hands. It's the heart that really does the healing" (p. 69). Healing permeates the story. As Ruggles helps wounded soldiers at Fort McPherson, she says, "I have more to offer than pity. I'm here to help these men" (p. 12). Others say of her, "She [has] an intense desire to help every one, to give freely and fully of her strength, her skills, her compassion and courage" (p. 63). She realizes that a significant part of helping means caring for each patient, and she acknowledges the cost:

> She and the other therapists had to fight to keep from becoming emotionally weakened by their atmosphere. If they turned hard, as many of the nurses did in self defense, they would lose the sensitivity and enthusiasm so necessary to their work. If they allowed themselves to be touched too deeply by the tragedy around them, they would become mentally disturbed—as, in fact, several young therapists did. (p. 77)

Ruggles maintains her sensitivity, as Major Benson acknowledges:

> The work that Miss Ruggles has accomplished here is little short of a miracle. . . . The camp has been transformed into a model of its kind. The men's morale has risen. Patients who had quite literally resigned themselves to death are more alive than ever. . . . (p. 130)

Ruggles describes an early insight into caring as she reflects about a particular patient:

> He hadn't done very well when I first started with him, but he's doing fine now. I asked myself why, and the answer suddenly came to me—the patient had improved because I had. I had become truly concerned about him. I wanted him to get well and I made him know I wanted him to get well. (p. 69)

Ruggles listens intently and understands her patients' values and goals. She responds by structuring activity options to meet the expressed needs of patients. She believes in the patient as primary healer. The story overflows with examples of Ruggles's responsiveness. One poignant example is her successful work with an angry and unruly patient who cannot tolerate sedentary crafts:

> "No, baskets aren't for you, Kilgore, and we both know it. I want you to make some spurs I've designed."
> His interest was immediately aroused. "Say, that sounds good. I used to be a cowboy you know. . . ."
> From the moment Kilgore went to work in the blacksmith shop, he never got into a fight. His gambling ceased entirely and he drank only moderately. After his discharge from the Army, he started an iron work plant which grew into one of the largest in the Southwest. (p. 91)

Ruggles describes her aim: "Most people have resources and reserves they don't even know about. My job, as I see it, is to bring out those resources and reserves. . . ." A captain responds, "Tell that to a man with no legs" (p. 52). Ruggles's rejoinder endorses the therapeutic caring specific to occupational therapy:

> "Oh, these aren't things you tell," Ora hastily explained. "These are things you do. The man with no legs would probably feel useless and unwanted . . . my problem is to get him to produce with his own hands something useful, beautiful or satisfying. . . . By personally making something useful, he feels useful—and wanted. He belongs." (p. 52)

Ruggles acknowledges personal gain from helping others: "I don't see what's missing, I see what's there. I see real manhood. I see great courage. I see tremendous strength. I see true spirit. That's what gives me courage, strength, and spirit. I gain as much or more as the men I try to help" (p. 76). Her sense of the mutuality in helping, her caring, and her competence enables her to help others.

One passage in *The Healing Heart* creates a lasting image. Paul, Ruggles's fiancé, tells her, "You're an artist in the greatest medium of all. You're an artist in people" (p. 92). She reflects that "it was indeed true that there was artistry in her work as a healer. She dealt with the soul, the heart and the spirit rather than paints and palette" (p. 92). The image the reader takes from this story is one of a therapist personally committed to each patient. This image is congruent with a vision of a personal relationship that balances competence in technique with caring in a relationship. Ruggles is a professional therapist; she is also a friend.

The Occupational Therapist as Technician, Parent, and Covenanter

Not all images of occupational therapists convey Ruggles's balance of competence and caring. Other stories present occupational therapists who seem bossy or preoccupied with crafts. One wonders how to characterize these images, how to begin to name them, in order to better understand and evaluate them. I have found it particularly helpful to turn to the writings of another person who thinks about professional relationships in terms of images.

May (1983) finds images helpful, both in clarifying functions and in establishing standards. He argues that "the image tells a kind of compressed story" (p. 17). An image is storylike in that it describes not only the basic character (in this case the physician), but also the person with whom the basic character interacts. If one thinks of a physician as a priest, for example, the priestly image suggests a relationship in which the physician is powerful and inspires awe in the patient. May (1983) discusses various images that he feels characterize physicians: three of the images— the technician, the parent, and the covenanter—seem relevant to this discussion of occupational therapy because they emerge from stories about occupational therapists. Technical occupational therapists are chiefly concerned with technique and technical issues, parental occupational therapists perceive and relate to their patients as dependents or children, and covenanting occupational therapists see their patients as bonded partners in the pursuit of therapeutic goals. Each of these images mirrors a markedly different understanding and manifestation of competence and caring.

The occupational therapist as technician. The therapist who functions as a technician commits to excellence in technical performance (May, 1983). Competence in technique preempts relationships; the therapist refines technical skills above all else. Although this image may seem cold, the basic impetus is humanitarian, because to the technical therapist only superior technical performance, efficiency, and use of correct procedure serve the patient's best interests. The occupational therapist whose primary focus is on methodology, percentage of function, or the task at hand is perceived by the patient as a technician.

In *No Laughing Matter* (Heller & Vogel, 1986), Heller describes his ordeal with Guillain-Barré syndrome and his experience with an occupational therapist who, though pleasant and humane, "possibly will be surprised or contrite to find out now of the very considerable anguish I experienced so often in my sessions with her or one of her co-workers" (p. 166). Methodology and gain are clearly important to this therapist:

> But in occupational therapy, as soon as I could sand a block of wood (with a need to rest both arms, it was written, after seven repetitions), a change was made to a coarser grade of sandpaper, increasing the amount of force required, and it was just as punishing and demoralizing for me to have to execute them as it had been in the beginning. (pp. 166–167)

Heller's overall impression is that "what they intended was to keep me always at a standstill" (p. 166). His personal need seems clear: to experience and then to savor a sense of gain. The therapist, oblivious to this need, implements a strategy to improve a condition. Treatment goals become the therapist's and clearly do not emanate from a collaborative relationship in which Heller's personal need has meaning.

Seabrook (1935) tells of his stay in a private mental institution for the treatment of his alcoholism. Although Seabrook's experience of occupational therapy is generally positive, he, too, views the occupational therapist as a technician. He describes one therapist/superintendent as "conscientious and probably having a kind heart, but nobody like[s] him" (p. 62). The superintendent values technique over relationship. Any personal or collaborative function that can be associated with occupational therapy rests with

Paschal, Seabrook's psychiatrist. Paschal mediates with the occupational therapist for different crafts and a more individualized approach to Seabrook. The occupational therapist provides competence; the psychiatrist provides care.

Another patient's story, this one in verse, portrays a predominantly technical occupational therapist. The opening lines introduce both the therapist and the elderly patient: "Preserve me from the occupational therapist, God. She means well, but I'm too busy to make baskets" (McClay, 1977, p. 106). The young therapist supports activity for its own sake. She makes no attempt to hear the patient or to discuss meaningful occupations; the patient–therapist exchanges merely parody the relationship:

> Oh, here she comes, the therapist, with
> scissors and paste.
> Would I like to try decoupage?
> "No," I say, "I haven't got time."
> "Nonsense," she says, "You're going to
> live a long, long time."
> That's not what I mean,
> I mean that all my life I've been
> doing things
> for people, with people. I have to
> catch up
> on my thinking and feeling. . . . (p. 107)

The concept of therapy as something that uses purposeful and meaningful activity to promote healing is predicated on some mutual understanding of personal meaning and interest. This therapist matches technique to patient type; she uses age, diagnosis, and disability to determine the choice of activity without regard for the patient's meaning and need. Activities chosen because protocol and the provider consider them meaningful may be reasonable forms of occupation, but they are questionable forms of occupational therapy.

The occupational therapist as parent. The image of parent is clearly a more personal one than that of detached technician. The parental image, typically associated with the provision of order and nurture, can be positive or negative depending on the manner in which order and nurture are provided (May, 1983). An excess of either order or nurture can compromise the relationship; helpers become paternalistic while patients become rebellious or dependent. The best parental figure, although excelling in knowledge and skill, bridges the power/knowledge gap through caring self-expenditure and compassion (May, 1983). I believe that he or she projects the positive image of a supportive parent who guards against exercising imbalance in the provision of order and nurture. The occupational therapist who threatens the patient's autonomy, rigidly and unilaterally enforces rules, or preempts the patient's decisions and fosters overdependence, however, conveys a negative parental image. Conversely, the therapist who supports the patient while trying to meet his or her need for order and nurture conveys a positive parental image.

The story of Brunhilde cited earlier illustrates the overauthoritative parent figure who wields power for the patient's own good (as defined by the therapist). Rule-bound Brunhilde eschews adult autonomy; caring, for her, is parenting gone awry. By contrast, Hanlan (1979) praises the parental occupational therapists who treated her husband:

> I was . . . impressed with the equanimity of occupational and physical therapists as they worked all day with severely handicapped people, some with terminal illnesses. . . . If helping personnel—social workers, physician, or whoever—conceived of their function with the terminally ill as helping with discrete, day-to-day problems, I believe they would have less trouble just "hanging in there," which is really the most essential ingredient. (p. 28)

The steadfastness of therapists who help patients with simple daily activities evokes a positive parental image.

The following fictional story about an activities therapist named Meg illustrates the parental therapist's vigilance against overnurture and overorder. Meg comes up with the idea of having patients in a private psychiatric hospital design and make living room drapes as a therapeutic activity. She benignly manipulates the patients into regarding the idea as their own, and they are enthusiastic about "their" project. The psychiatrist later commends her for her skillful handling of the situation. She acknowledges that it was "handling" and questions the appropriateness of her conduct. Her psychiatrist friend answers:

> I don't think you did any—violence to their being; the idea was in them or you couldn't have wooed it out. And dealing with patients always takes some handling, the question is only is it for their benefit or yours. (Gibson, 1979, p. 51)

The psychiatrist's rationalization for this benignly paternalistic intervention is typical: The intervention is justifiable if it is for the patient's own good.

The occupational therapist as covenanter. May's (1983) image of the occupational therapist as covenanter illustrates a relationship equivalent to friendship. A friend (as covenanter) acknowledges an element of gift in human relationships. For one who covenants with another, a sense of reciprocity characterizes the giving and receiving. The professional steeped in the spirit of covenant regards his professional skills as gifts to be shared with a community of others. Services rendered occur within the context of a trusted relationship, and both parties receive as well as give. Although reciprocity characterizes the relationship within a covenanted bond, the stronger partner uses strengths and skills to nourish and build up the weaker (May, 1983). Above all, the friend, as covenanted person, professes commitment to the patient, based on personal respect. Within the context of this friendship, the therapist collaborates and cooperates with the patient's self-actualization. Petersen (1976) describes a way of collaborating in self-actualization that includes activity. It could well represent an occupational therapist who is a friend:

> There is a shouting spirit deep inside me:
> Take clay, it cries,
> Take pen and ink,
> Take flour and water,
> Take a scrub brush,
> Take a yellow crayon
> Take another's hand
> And with all these
>   Say you,
>   Say loving.

Certainly the image of Ora Ruggles from *The Healing Heart* is that of a friend. Other patients' stories also portray occupational therapists as friends: Benziger (1969) tells of her hospitalization for depression, remembering the occupational therapist as her "new friend" (p. 48). She notes her first impression of the therapist:

> A few days later the first person I had met there who made any real sense came into my room. She was the occupational therapist—a term I've always hated. She was kind, interested, enthusiastic, full of ideas, and intelligent. (p. 47)

The occupational therapist trusts Benziger, follows through on promises made, and supports a desire to get well. Crafts serve as catalysts for their interactions about life. The following exchange shows how the occupational therapist is responsive to Benziger and respects her strengths:

> "You know, you go at your work too hard, too fast, too desperately—and too frenetically."
>
> "I guess I do, but that's the way I feel. Time stands still for me now, it is endless, and yet if I have something to do, I get the sense that there will not be time enough to finish it, or that someone will stop me. . . ."
>
> She said, "You are an intelligent person, and you will help yourself to get well quickly."
>
> "You know," I answered, "you're the first person who has mentioned intelligence versus non intelligence, instead of sanity. You make me feel like a human being. . . ." I was grateful. I should not forget her. (p. 49)

A third image of occupational therapist as friend appears in Donaldson's (1976) autobiographical account of his unwanted and unwarranted 15-year confinement in mental institutions. That Donaldson could, under the circumstances, perceive any staff as friendly comes as a surprise. Nonetheless, Donaldson considers the occupational therapy worker, Baldylocks, a friend:

> While I waited, I found OT fun. Young, overweight Baldylocks had about five of us. He was a zealous worker in his church, and did not swear, drink, or smoke. He translated his religion to his work by showing compassion and understanding to all of us. He let me spend afternoons learning the touch

> system of typing. . . . Baldylocks started taking the OT men and a half dozen from upstairs for a two-hour walk on the grounds each Wednesday. Under the umbrella of all this warmth, I began watching the news on TV again. (pp. 245–246)

In occupational therapy, Donaldson exercises, cooks, and learns lathe work—all fulfilling activities selected in a spirit of collaboration and cooperation. Donaldson sees clearly this occupational therapy worker's commitment to caring, trust, and respect.

Patients' stories, then, suggest that occupational therapists can project an image of technician, parent, or friend, because therapists understand the therapeutic relationship in different ways. Images from patients' stories mirror the manner in which various patients experienced demonstrations of therapists' competence and caring.

Variable Emphases on Competence and Caring

Patients' positive images of occupational therapists reflect both competence and caring. Negative images reflect either a failure to commit personally to care or competence or caring gone awry. May's images are helpful both in characterizing occupational therapists and in understanding various interpretations of the occupational therapy vision of relationship. Each of May's three images—technician, parent, and friend—emphasizes competence and caring in a slightly different way. For the technical therapist, competence in performance is the primary expression of caring. Personal investment in the patient stimulates the pursuit of excellence in technique. The positive parental therapist, on the other hand, demonstrates caring, but the caring is powerful; the therapist must guard against falling into handling or managing the patient. Unlike the technician, for whom competence is assumed to be caring, a parental therapist's care presumes competence. The parental caregiver determines how care should be given. Although many patients value care, they challenge the assumption that the caregiver always knows best. The therapist-as-friend image works to resolve the caring–competence struggle found in parental and technical images by assigning equal value to both care and competence. A therapist who would be a friend to the patient commits to competence and caring because the patient is a person who deserves both.

Although there will always be individual patients who want therapists to function as technicians or parents, many patients and occupational therapists call for a different image, one that equalizes competence and caring and that generates images of occupational therapists as friends. Public distress over impersonal care has resulted in a series of measures to acknowledge patients' rights: quality assurance requirements, the Patient's Bill of Rights, informed consent legislation, and the regulation of experimentation on human beings. These measures create a systematic defense against a powerful and technologically advanced medical system that tends to depersonalize the individual patient. The health care system demands scientific and technical competence; the legal system demands the acknowledgment of individual rights. Practitioners must be competent to function in the health care system without creating a service that is devoid of caring. Commitment to caring about a person cannot be legislated; it can, however, be part of a profession's vision.

Hodgins (1969) powerfully describes his post-stroke experiences in his article, "Whatever Became of the Healing Art?" He mourns the loss of the family physician who "was a friend to his patients, one function among many others which most of today's practitioners have completely given up" (p. 838). He values occupational therapists who "have so much more a satisfactory grasp on the real needs of the stroke patient" (p. 841). Hodgins wonders about the patient in today's health care system:

> From whom, then, is he to draw the courage without which he will not truly recover? Not from a silent practitioner; not from a stuffy practitioner; not from a practitioner, whether doctor, therapist, or nurse, who is aloof. He will draw courage as he perceives human understanding underlying the professional techniques of those into whose care he has been given. (p. 841)

In 1980, several therapists addressed the concept of caring at the 60th Annual Conference of the American Occupational Therapy Association. Together their remarks echoed those of Hodgins; they endorsed a vision of the therapeutic relationship that approximates that of pioneer Ora Ruggles, that of the therapist as friend. At the heart of this vision is the belief that the patient–therapist relationship is integral to practice. Baum (1980) writes, "We are nothing more than a bystander in the life of [the patient] until a relationship is formed" (p. 514). Competence and caring remain key elements in the vision, but both are effective only insofar as they reflect sensitive commitment to a patient who is first of all a person. Activity selection and treatment goals must have personal meaning for the patient; meaningful choice is essential because it fosters personal control. Baum (1980) clarifies the process: "Occupational therapy harnesses will and gives the individual control through activity. That is human, that is care" (p. 515). Technical skills work only within the context of a relationship: "Skills promote movement and flexibility within our therapeutic relationships. . . . Skills in caring provide us with the ability to modify the technique according to another person's needs" (Gilfoyle, 1980,

p. 520). King (1980) identifies the commitment to caring that must permeate competence: "Occupational therapy is one of the 'helping' professions, with the assumption that help is the outgrowth of caring" (p. 522). Competence must be rooted in caring for a person.

Caring also needs to be rooted in commitment to the patient as a person. Gilfoyle (1980) writes:

> The caring therapist directly knows a client as a unique individual, as someone in his or her own right, not as an average, a generality, or a number on the Gaussian curve. . . . Implicit knowledge is the art of "being with the person"; it is something you feel. (p. 520)

The person is experienced and respected as an "other" with strengths and capabilities; "the 'caring' is not the taking-care-of the person, but helping the person learn to take care of himself/herself" (Gilfoyle, 1980, p. 519). The same principle can be stated in another way: "Through our professional relationships we reach out and with empathy show that we care hoping that from this caring . . . the person will find his or her own strength" (Baum, 1980, p. 515).

Yerxa (1980) regards deliberations on caring as calibrations of the profession's success. She says, "Our practice in the future should be evaluated not only on the basis of measurable scientific outcomes, but also by what it contributes to individual human dignity, a sense of mastery and self-respect" (p. 534). She identifies the challenge of the future as that of preserving and embracing a climate of caring "in the face of a society increasingly dominated by technique and objectivism" (p. 532). This type of caring resembles a friendship in which "patient and therapist enter into a partnership, and in which patients have the authority to determine their own needs" (p. 532).

Conclusion

The vision of the therapeutic relationship in occupational therapy has, despite its evolving emphasis and sometimes fragmentary form, encompassed two essential features: competence and caring. Images that patients have held of occupational therapists have varied, partly because of the ways in which therapists have understood and acted on their understanding of how to balance competence and caring during their interactions with patients. Negative images of occupational therapists found in patients' stories suggest that therapists who present themselves primarily as technicians or parents are more apt to disappoint the patient.

A health care system that depersonalizes patients challenges occupational therapists to assess the vision of the therapeutic relationship that has inspired their practice. Recommitment to regarding the patient as a vital partner—as a friend—can lead to exchanges marked by mutuality, caring, and competence. Commitment to a balance of technical competence and personal caring, for the sake of a friend, can shape a healing image. ▲

Acknowledgments

I thank Sally Gadow, PhD, and Anne Hudson Jones, PhD, of the Institute for the Medical Humanities, University of Texas Medical Branch at Galveston, for their encouragement and suggestions. I also thank Paula Levine, School of Allied Health Sciences, University of Texas Medical Branch, for her editorial suggestions.

References

Baum, C. (1980). Occupational therapists put care in the health system. *American Journal of Occupational Therapy, 34,* 505–516.

Benziger, B. (1969). *The prison of my mind.* New York: Walker.

Carlova, J., & Ruggles, O. (1946). *The healing heart.* New York: Messner.

Donaldson, K. (1976). *Insanity inside out.* New York: Crown.

Fay, E. V., & March, I. (1947). Occupational therapy in general and special hospitals. In H. S. Willard & C. S. Spackman (Eds.), *Principles of occupational therapy* (pp. 118–137). Philadelphia: J. B. Lippincott.

Gibson, W. (1979). *The cobweb.* New York: Atheneum Press.

Gilfoyle, E. (1980). Caring: A philosophy of practice. *American Journal of Occupational Therapy, 34,* 517–521.

Gleave, G. M. (1947). Occupational therapy in children's hospitals and pediatric services. In H. S. Willard & C. S. Spackman (Eds.), *Principles of occupational therapy* (pp. 141–174). Philadelphia: J. B. Lippincott.

Hanlan, M. (1979, November). Living with a dying husband. *Pennsylvania Gazette,* pp. 25–28.

Heller, J., & Vogel, S. (1986). *No laughing matter.* New York: Avon.

Hodgins, E. (1969). Whatever became of the healing art? *Annals of the New York Academy of Sciences, 164,* 838–846.

Hopkins, H. L., & Smith, H. D. (Eds.). (1983). *Willard and Spackman's occupational therapy* (6th ed.). Philadelphia: J. B. Lippincott.

Hopkins, H. L., & Tiffany, E. G. (1983). Occupational therapy—A problem-solving process. In H. L. Hopkins & H. D. Smith (Eds.), *Willard and Spackman's occupational therapy* (6th ed., pp. 89–100). Philadelphia: J. B. Lippincott.

King, L. J. (1980). Creative caring. *American Journal of Occupational Therapy, 34,* 522–528.

May, W. (1983). *The physician's covenant: Images of the healer in medical ethics.* Philadelphia: Westminster Press.

McClay, E. (1977). *Green winter: Celebrations of old age.* New York: Reader's Digest Press.

Peloquin, S. M. (1989). Sustaining the art of occupational therapy. *American Journal of Occupational Therapy, 43,* 219–226.

Petersen, J. (1976). *A book of yes.* Illinois: Argus Communications.

Purtilo, R. (1978). *Health professional/patient interaction.* Philadelphia: W. B. Saunders.

Rebeta-Burditt, J. (1977). *The cracker factory.* New York: Bantam.

Seabrook, W. (1935). *Asylum.* New York: Harcourt, Brace.

Smith, H. D., & Tiffany, E. G. (1983). Assessment and evaluation—An overview. In H. L. Hopkins & H. D. Smith (Eds.), *Willard and Spackman's occupational therapy* (6th ed., pp. 143–148). Philadelphia: J. B. Lippincott.

Tiffany, E. G. (1983). Psychiatry and mental health. In H. L. Hopkins & H. D. Smith (Eds.), *Willard and Spackman's occupational therapy* (6th ed., pp. 267–329). Philadelphia: J. B. Lippincott.

Wade, B. D. (1947). Occupational therapy for patients with mental disease. In H. S. Willard & C. S. Spackman (Eds.), *Principles of occupational therapy* (pp. 81–117). Philadelphia: J. B. Lippincott.

Willard, H. S., & Spackman, C. S. (Eds.). (1947). *Principles of occupational therapy.* Philadelphia: J. B. Lippincott.

Yerxa, E. J. (1980). Occupational therapy's role in creating a future climate of caring. *American Journal of Occupational Therapy, 34,* 529–534.

Sustaining the Art of Practice in Occupational Therapy

Suzanne M. Peloquin

Key Words: caregivers • human activities
and occupation • literature • patient
advocacy • professional–patient relations

The art of practice in occupational therapy is intrinsically centered on relationships, on the qualities that make relationships meaningful, and on the meaning of occupation in a life. Demands from today's health care system make it increasingly difficult for practitioners to engage in meaningful relationships with their patients. The art of practice, jeopardized by the health care system, requires sustenance from other sources. A new field, literature and medicine, suggests a source of sustenance for the art of occupational therapy practice. The reading of fictional literature can provide occupational therapists with sustaining images that can reaffirm their commitment to the art of providing occupation as therapy.

Suzanne M. Peloquin, MA, OTR, is Assistant Professor, School of Allied Health Sciences, The University of Texas Medical Branch, Galveston, Texas 77551.

This article was accepted for publication June 12, 1988.

Occupational therapists have seen an effort within their profession to unearth historical roots, to articulate a philosophical base, to elucidate models for practice, and to validate theoretical concepts through research. The search for a professional identity and for professional credibility is essential; it has also been intense. The purpose of this article is to explore a concept that has been underrepresented in occupational therapy literature over the last decade: the art of the practice of occupational therapy.

The art of occupational therapy is the soul of its practice. Therapy as an art is an old theme; literature as a nurturer of the soul is an older theme still. The occupational therapy literature with its many references to paradigms, constructs, and variables reflects a considerable effort to articulate the profession's scientific basis. A profession committed to balance can perhaps sustain its art by reflecting on the images of caring and helpful occupation seen in fictional literature.

The Art of Occupational Therapy

In 1972, the American Occupational Therapy Association (AOTA) Council on Standards defined occupational therapy as "the art and science of directing man's participation in selected tasks to restore, reinforce and enhance performance, facilitate learning of those skills and functions essential for adaptation and productivity, diminish or correct pathology, and to promote and maintain health" (p. 204). Years later, AOTA's Representative Assembly accepted a more comprehensive definition that begins as follows:

> Occupational therapy is the use of purposeful activity with individuals who are limited by physical injury or illness, psychosocial dysfunction, developmental or learning disabilities, poverty and cultural differences or aging process in order to maximize independence, prevent disability and maintain health. (1981, p. 798)

Definitions evolve over time to reflect changes in priorities and orientations. It is not surprising that the descriptive phrase "art and science," which validates a blend of practice components, was deleted between 1972 and 1981 as the profession's emphasis turned toward scientific research and accountability.

In spite of this deletion from the profession's official definition, the practice of occupational therapy remains a blend of art and science. There is an art to the practice of any therapeutic endeavor. Mosey (1981) discussed art relative to the practice of occupational therapy. She first defined the art of practice negatively, stating that the art of practice is not (a) a desire to help others, (b) the skilled application of scientific knowledge, or (c) simply being a systematic or sympathetic practitioner. Mosey wrote, "The capacity to establish rapport, to empathize, and to guide others to know and make use of their potential as participants in a community of others illustrates the art of occupational therapy" (p. 4). Without art, she claimed, occupational therapy would become the application of scientific knowledge in a sterile vacuum.

Mosey (1981) elaborated those characteristics commonly held by practitioners she called "masters in the art of practice" (p. 23). The artful practitioner perceives the individual as indivisible into various parts or subsystems. Although practitioners reduce the human organism into subsystems in order to understand the patient more clearly, the art of practice reintegrates those subsystems to see a whole person. Meeting the patient as an individual enables the practitioner to empathize with the patient and to accept his or her feelings, ideas, and values. The meaning that the patient places on his or her life, relationships, and environment guides the therapist–patient collaboration toward growth, independence, and the use of potential.

The science of practice, Mosey (1981) said, is a phenomenon fundamental to all professions. In occupational therapy practice, science is the gathering of data through systematic clinical observations or through more formalized research projects to help develop new theories or to verify, refine, or refute existing theories relevant to the practice. The art and the science of occupational therapy together constitute its practice.

Devereaux (1984) identified the caring relationship as the art rather than the science of health care. She wrote, "Occupational therapists are specialists in making care happen. We know how to enrich all the transactions in the relationship with the patient. These become caring gestures" (p. 794). Devereaux characterized the particular caring of occupational therapists as singular among professionals: helping the patient reconnect to those occupations that are meaningful to him or her. She said, "Occupational therapists care by helping people disengage from despair and dysfunction and by helping them look forward, to see their loss as being able to be ameliorated through adaptation and occupation" (p. 794).

Within the context of her definition of caring, Devereaux (1984) highlighted a major assumption that informs the theory and the practice of occupational therapy: that adaptation occurs through the use of occupation. According to Reed and Sanderson (1983), occupational therapy theory and practice build on several assumptions. Although it is difficult to summarize these assumptions, Reed and Sanderson demonstrated that it is possible. They categorized a long list that included assumptions about: (a) human beings; (b) occupational performance; (c) health, wellness, and illness; (d) the receipt of health care services; (e) the provision of health care; (f) occupa-

tional therapy; and (g) the therapeutic use of occupations. In the art of practice, as occupational therapists engage meaningfully with patients, they discuss assumptions. They formulate treatment plans based on mutual assumptions chosen from among several possible categories. A cluster of assumptions gleaned from Reed and Sanderson's comprehensive list seems central to the caring connection described by Devereaux. These assumptions relate to occupation and figure prominently in any dialogue with patients about their connection with meaningfulness:

> Each individual must perform some occupation or have the occupations performed for the person to survive.
> A person adapts or adjusts (grows and develops) through the use of and participation in various occupations.
> Occupations may be divided into three major areas: self-maintenance, productivity and leisure.
> A balance of occupations is facilitatory to the maintenance of a satisfying life.
> Occupations permit a person to fulfill individual and group needs.
> Occupations must be relevant and useful to the individual in relating to the environment. (p. 70)

The art of practice supports the entire structure of occupational therapy. Caring, informed by assumptions about occupation, constitutes the base for those elements Devereaux (1984) considered essential to an effective relationship in occupational therapy: (a) competence, (b) belief in the dignity and worth of the person, (c) belief that each person has the potential for change and growth, (d) communication, (e) values, (f) touch, and (g) sense of humor. Caring transforms a science of occupation into a therapeutic practice.

Mastery of the art of practice in the fullness described by Mosey (1981) and Devereaux (1984) is a challenge. One need only reflect on the current demands faced by practitioners to acknowledge the difficulty. The brief length of patients' stays, the demands for productivity, the documentation criteria for third-party reimbursers and accrediting agencies, and the requirements for research and quality assurance all demand the time and energy required for caring. Occupational therapy practitioners need affirmation that the art of practice is valued and that those assumptions about occupation that are communicated through caring are relevant to patients. Today's health care system does not tend to nurture the art; it does not encourage consistent patient–therapist dialogue about assumptions.

Associates of occupational therapy in medicine have been vocal in their articulation of the struggle to retain the humane side of practice. Engel (1977) wrote of physicians' disenchantment with an approach to disease that neglects the patient, with a dominance of procedures over patient sensitivities, and with a biomedical emphasis that disregards human meaning. Pellegrino (1979) claimed that the concepts of discreteness of disease processes and specificity of therapeutic agents have transformed the ethos of medicine. Therapeutics as we know it today, a little more than a century old, has been beneficial for humankind on the whole. But the impact of scientific advances and technological successes has profoundly compromised the relationship between patient and physician.

Patients resent the fragmentation of their care. Public distress has resulted in a series of measures to acknowledge the patient, the person, and his or her rights: quality assurance, the patient's bill of rights, legal concern with informed consent, and the regulation of experimentation on human beings. These measures systematize a defense against a powerful medical system that tends to forget or ignore the individual patient. The health care system demands scientific competence; the legal system demands acknowledgment of individual rights. There is no escaping the reality: Practitioners must engage in the science of practice in order to function in the health care system. And yet, patients and professionals alike recognize the sterility of a human service practice devoid of its art, its caring. Rights can be legislated, but caring cannot. The art of practice, not so valued or nurtured by the health care system, requires sustenance from other sources.

Literature: Toward an Affirmation of the Art of Practice

A new field, literature and medicine, suggests a source of sustenance for the art of occupational therapy practice. Jones (1987) characterized literature and medicine as a recent phase in the medical humanities experiment in medical education. She identified two approaches to literature that justify its incorporation into medical education: the aesthetic and the moral. Trautmann (1978) described the aesthetic approach: "to teach a student to read, in the fullest sense" (p. 36). The fictional world, she said, reveals "relationships between people and within a single personality" (p. 33). In reading fiction, one "must look at words in their personal and social contexts" (p. 36). Trautmann said that through literature one can make the leap to empathy, to compassion. Through literature, one can achieve affirmation of personal dignity—affirmation of a personhood threatened by the health care system.

Coles (1979), a physician, described the second approach to literature, the moral approach. He wrote that "the point of a medical humanities course devoted to literature is ethical reflection" (p. 445). Coles believed that novelists and clinicians alike focus on the everyday life and on the unique nature of the human being. He said that there is a continuing tension between one's idealism and life's demands.

Novelists, he said, can move one to scrutinize assumptions, expectations, and values, to reflect on a life either as it is being lived or as one hopes to live it.

Images from fictional literature viewed within the context of either the aesthetic or the moral approach can nurture the art of occupational therapy practice. The art of practice, is, after all, intrinsically centered on images—images of relationships, of qualities that make relationships meaningful, of occupation's meaning in a life.

The aesthetic approach to literature can help, in its scrutiny of relationships, to validate the meaningfulness of "the capacity to establish rapport, to empathize, and to guide others to know and make use of their potential as participants in a community of others" (Mosey, 1981, p. 4). The moral approach can prompt reflection about practice elements and about assumptions that inform practice. Both approaches can validate the practitioner's commitment to the art, to caring, and to caring connections.

Yerxa and Sharrott (1986), in their endorsement of a liberal arts education for occupational therapists, wrote

> Occupational therapy's knowledge base requires an understanding of medical conditions, but it is not the medical condition per se that is of the greatest significance; rather, it is the occupational nature of the human being. Thus, although our knowledge, in practice, is primarily applied to people who are ill and disabled, the science of occupation and its concern with the play–work continuum, adaptation, and competence development applies to all people, disabled or not. (p. 158)

Literature, read in its fullest sense and reflected upon, can contribute to an understanding of the human condition.

Mosey (1981) described the process of learning the art of practice: "The individual who strives to bring art to practice must be able to engage in the often uncomfortable process of learning more about one's self, changing one's self, and gaining knowledge about how one's values and expectations may differ from those of others" (p. 25). In the world of fiction one can find a mirror reflecting back, for recognition and appraisal, one's self, one's values, and one's expectations. One can also find in the world of fiction a window opening onto a world of others, their values, and their expectations. Literature can facilitate learning the art of practice.

Fiction: A Reflection of the Art of Practice

The concept of reading fiction to enhance the art of practice will no doubt elicit varied responses from widely diverse occupational therapy practitioners. Avid, discriminating readers use the process already, but nonreaders may not be intrinsically motivated to turn to fiction without a clear indication that the process can enhance their skill in the art of practice. Although the process seems particularly suited to the educational system, it is equally adaptable to any continued learning endeavor.

The fictional world is populated by occupational therapists and patients. Some images from that world reflect practitioners inept in the art of practice and patients vocal about that ineptitude. Fiction also contains images that seriously challenge assumptions about occupation. If one expects sustenance from the literature, one needs to know how to handle the negative images.

Reading in a fuller sense can be affirming, even if the fictionalized occupational therapist happens to be a rogue or a villain. If one can agree that the character's interpersonal style lacks care, that agreement affirms one's endorsement of a different style: "I'll be (or I am) a different kind of occupational therapist." This can be affirming. Reading in the fuller sense, one can find other characters whose interactional styles are favorably represented. To reflect on characteristics worth emulating is to once again affirm one's belief in caring and in the art of practice.

An encounter in the fictional world with a blatant repudiation of an assumption about occupational therapy may be disturbing. By reading in the moral sense, that is, reading to examine human values, one can step out of one's own world of assumptions to consider those of others. This experience can enrich later dialogues with patients. The exploration of another world through fiction can enable one to better understand real patients whose values differ from one's own. The reflection and the broadening of view made possible through fiction can facilitate the meeting of each patient as an individual.

In *The Cracker Factory* (Rebeta-Burditt, 1977), an occupational therapist working in a private psychiatric hospital is characterized in a most unflattering manner. The protagonist in this story is Cassie, a young woman admitted to the hospital because she is depressed and abusing alcohol. Cassie does not single the occupational therapist out for criticism; the therapist is one of several characters seen as oppressive. Cassie describes her hospital experiences satirically. She depicts the occupational therapist in an interactionally challenging scene: attempting to motivate patients to come to a therapy group. Cassie names the therapist "Brunhilde, the misplaced Viking Lady" and "the Dictator of OT" (p. 114). Both names suggest an abuse of power. One expects ferocious and bloody battle with a Viking and arbitrary orders from a dictator. The names, unfortunately, seem apt. The therapist "marches around the seventh floor telling all the patients that their doctor has 'ordered' Occupational Therapy" (p. 114). Rather than discussing with individual patients the merits of therapy or its relevance to them personally, she invokes the power of the doctor's order. She "herds them out in the hall"

and "goosesteps them out the door" (p. 114). There is no evidence of rapport here, no humor, no recognition of patients as individuals. Harshness dominates the scene.

The occupational therapist insists that the patients "must come IMMEDIATELY" (p. 114). When patients try to hide from her by taking a shower, "She doesn't care. Wet or screaming, it makes no difference. She drags them along anyway" (pp. 114–115). A caring touch is replaced by dragging and goose-stepping. Notably absent are a respect for patients' dignity and an acknowledgment of patients' rights. There is clearly no empathy. Instead, there are threats: "If you don't go to OT, it will be written down on your chart and you won't get out of here" (p. 114). Cassie's perception of the motivational attempt is one of intimidation. The reader is forced to agree.

Practitioners may recognize in this portrayal the familiar struggle inherent in the motivational process. Ultimately, the patient has the right to refuse all treatment, for whatever reason. Furthermore, the patient has every right to dispute or to reject any and all assumptions about the therapeutic process. Meanwhile, the concerned practitioner, invested in the patient as a person, tries to communicate possible benefits, to convey a deep personal interest, to attempt to collaborate, and to walk away from the motivational effort only when convinced that the patient has sufficient information to have made a real choice.

Powerful images from *The Cracker Factory* stimulate reflection about the motivational attempt. Does even the best attempt feel, to the patient, like a battle? If so, what interpersonal elements might signal a truce? Cassie's view clearly reminds therapists that a patient who has little control over an environment perceives those in control as dictators. What therapist characteristics might impress a patient differently? *The Cracker Factory* provides a clue to anyone reading in the fuller sense.

One favorite nurse escapes Cassie's sharp criticism: the nurse she calls Tinkerbell. Tink does not invoke rules or orders. She makes exceptions to the rules when possible. Cassie comes in from the cold, after a late-night Alcoholics Anonymous meeting, and Tink tosses her a set of keys saying, "The kitchen is officially closed but you may go in if you like" (p. 221). Cassie is "delighted, feeling like a friend" (p. 221). Tink takes time to establish rapport, to be with Cassie, to talk with her. She asks personal questions, and she encourages Cassie to share. When Cassie says of herself, "I doubt I'll ever have the ability to be that open," Tink says, "Give it time. . . . When you're more comfortable, you'll loosen up" (p. 222). When Cassie asks Tink a personal question, Tink agrees to answer, saying, "Okay, Cassie, I'll play fair" (p. 223). She shares a personally painful situation. Unlike

Brunhilde, whom Cassie describes as not caring, Cassie tells Tink, "You care," to which Tink nods and replies, "I care" (p. 227). But Tink admits personal shortcomings. She says, "I have limitations like everyone else" (p. 227). She tells Cassie, "I prefer involvement on a limited basis, caring on my terms, the way I handle it best, the way I'm most effective" (p. 227). Tink's disclosure of personal weaknesses has therapeutic value. She can say, "Cassie . . . from where I'm standing, I have a clear view of *your* strengths" (p. 227). Tink's display of humanity reinforces Cassie's humanity. In Cassie's worldview, Tink is a caring person; the occupational therapist is not. The art in Tink's practice of nursing contrasts harshly with the absence of art in the occupational therapist's practice.

Interactional characteristics make a difference to patients in fiction and in reality. The exaggeration and striking contrast between one occupational therapist and one nurse used in *The Cracker Factory* can generate powerful responses and productive thinking. The kind of reflection that is prompted by an encounter with forceful fictional characters can nurture the art of practice.

Images of Occupation and Caring Connections

In addition to specific images of occupational therapists in literature, there are images of occupation and of caring people associated with occupation. Two literary pieces, Kesey's *One Flew Over the Cuckoo's Nest* (1962) and Shem's *The House of God* (1978), have achieved a measure of notoriety for their portrayals of health care environments in which professional caring is painfully compromised.

Kesey's novel depicts a state mental institution. The story is told from the point of view of the Chief, an electively mute, chronically ill American Indian patient. The Chief's delusional system and active visual and auditory hallucinations contribute to the image that patients are caught in a gigantic unyielding machine designed to socialize them into conformity. The typical hospital day is monotonous: Acutes and Chronics alike submit to the order imposed by the Big Nurse. The Chief describes the atmosphere: "There's something strange about a place where the men won't let themselves loose and laugh, something strange about the way they all knuckle under to that smiling flour-faced old mother [Big Nurse]" (p. 48). He describes group discussion among the patients as "telling things that wouldn't ever let them look one another in the eye again" (p. 49). He characterizes the therapies offered as being all the same and unable to engage the patient: "Ten-forty, -forty-five, -fifty, patients shuttle in and out to appointments in ET or OT or PT" (p. 38). The environment is devoid of meaningful occupation and meaningful interpersonal exchange; the result is dehumanizing.

Shem describes an equally maladaptive environment in *The House of God*. Roy Basch is an intern at the House of God, a hospital where the "emphasis was on doing everything always for everyone forever to keep the patient alive" (pp. 25–26). The House of God is filled with gomers, "human beings who have lost what goes into being human beings" (p. 38). Within this environment, interns and residents lack support from their supervisors, struggle against exhaustion, and grapple with life, death, and ethical issues. Tired interns focus on getting sleep: "I wish she would die so I could just go to sleep" (p. 135). They try to learn "enough medicine to worry less about saving patients and more about saving [them]selves" (p. 150). They always seem on the edge of sanity and control. Roy says, "I'm scared that one of these nights, with nobody else around, when someone starts to abuse me, I'm going to lose control and beat the shit out of some poor bastard" (pp. 232–233). There is no balance of occupations, no rest, and no leisure. Roy describes his inner state at his worst point: "I had been as far from the world of humans as I could get. . . . I had been sarcastic. I'd avoided feeling everything, as if feelings were little grenades" (p. 361). Roy Basch, denied a balance of occupations and cut off from meaningful human exchange by the demands and stresses of work, lives in an environment as dehumanized as that portrayed by the Chief.

Kesey and Shem provide hope for both the Chief and Roy Basch: there is a way out of these maladaptive environments and these dehumanizing worlds. Other people lead the way out, people who can laugh, who can relate, who can touch. People help the Chief and Roy to make connections with helpful occupations.

In *One Flew Over the Cuckoo's Nest*, McMurphy enters the Chief's world: "He sounds big. I hear him coming down the hall, and he sounds big in the way he walks. . . . He talks a little the way Papa used to, voice loud and full of hell" (p. 16). McMurphy laughs. The Chief says, "I realize all of a sudden it's the first laugh I've heard in years" (p. 16). McMurphy's activity level is contagious. He plays cards and Monopoly, he pitches pennies, he commandeers a tub room for a game room, he socializes and gambles incessantly, he struggles with Big Nurse over the use of the TV. The longer McMurphy stays, the more in touch with reality the Chief becomes. McMurphy organizes two activities (or occupations) in particular that seem to make meaningful connections for others: a basketball game on the ward and a fishing trip.

McMurphy "talk[s] the doctor into letting him bring a ball back from the gym" (p. 174). In response to the nurse's objections, the doctor observes: "A number of the players, Miss Ratched, have shown marked progress since that basketball team was organized; I think it has proven its therapeutic value" (p.

175). The team increases a feeling of solidarity among the patients. The Chief, though not on the team, says, "We got to go to the gym and watch our basketball team" (p. 176). The game "let most of [them] come away feeling there'd been a kind of victory" (p. 176) despite their 20-point loss. The image of this patients' team is familiar to most occupational therapists: "Our team was too short and too slow, and Martini kept throwing passes to men that nobody but him could see" (p. 176). The adaptive effects represented in this image of the game validate a major occupational therapy assumption about the human condition.

When basketball season is over, McMurphy plans a fishing trip. He deceives authorities into thinking that two maiden aunts will sponsor the expedition. Instead, he engages the help of a prostitute. The Chief focuses his attention increasingly on McMurphy's energy and strength. When he speaks for the first time in years, he speaks to McMurphy. After having been withdrawn for years, the Chief yearns to reach out. He thinks, "I just want to touch him because he's who he is" (p. 188). McMurphy signs the Chief up for the fishing trip. The Chief reflects: "I was actually going out of the hospital with two whores on a fishing boat; I had to keep saying it over and over to myself to believe it" (p. 191).

Images of the fishing trip powerfully present the competence, mastery, and connectedness with others possible through occupation. The activity meets both group and individual needs. The trip is an occupation enjoyable to these men both in the doing and in the end product: the successful catch. Fiction here validates on a dramatic level what a formal analysis might predict about this particular activity for a group of institutionalized patients. Each person on the expedition benefits in some way from the activity. The Chief's experience is representative of that of the others. On the ride he says, "I could feel a great calmness creep over me, a calmness that increased the farther we left land behind us" (p. 208). He recalls that he "was as excited as the rest" (p. 209). He fishes independently: "I was too busy cranking at my fish to ask him [McMurphy] for help" (p. 210). The clearest representation of the healing effect of the experience is the spread of McMurphy's laughter. The Chief says, "I notice Harding is collapsed beside McMurphy and is laughing too. And Scanlon from the bottom of the boat . . . . It started slow and pumped itself full, swelling the men bigger and bigger. I watched, part of them, laughing with them" (p. 212). The Chief explains that McMurphy knows about laughter: "He knows you have to laugh at the things that hurt you just to keep yourself in balance, just to keep the world from running you plumb crazy" (p. 212). From within the context of a dehumanizing state institution, a real

person, capable of relating and capable of touching lives, makes connections for these men using occupations that help them heal. This image can nurture the art of occupational therapy practice.

In *The House of God,* Roy Basch's experience cuts him off from a number of caring peers. Two people manage to help Roy reconnect through occupations. Roy's girlfriend, Berry, quietly reflects back to him the changes she sees. Toward the end of the novel she says, "Roy, I'm worried. . . . You're isolated. . . . You're hypomanic. . . . For me, tonight, you're a dead man. There's no spark of life" (p. 349). She organizes a trip to see a performance of the mime Marcel Marceau. Roy tries to get out of going at the last minute, so Berry has four of Roy's friends literally carry him out of the hospital to the performance. Seeing the mime perform, Roy reflects, "All of a sudden I felt as if a hearing aid for all my senses had been turned on. I was flooded with feeling" (p. 359). Later he says, "Berry welcomed me back to her, and I felt her caring arms around me for the first time. Awakening, I began to thaw" (p. 360). The performance, in its dramatic portrayal of the human struggle, touches Roy and reconnects him with his innermost self. He says, "I realized that what had been missing [from the House of God experience] was all that I loved. I would be transformed. I'd not leave that country of love again" (p. 363). Soon after the performance, Roy describes his internship: "I hated this. The whole year sucked" (p. 374). Berry asks him, "Why not become a psychiatrist? . . . Being with people was all that kept you going this year, Roy. And 'being with' is the essence of psychiatry" (p. 374). Berry, having connected Roy to a powerful experience that enabled him to feel again, suggests an occupation in which his need to feel and care might be allowed to grow. This healing image is also one that validates the art of occupational therapy practice.

The Fat Man is a caring resident in *The House of God.* In some ways a renegade like Kesey's McMurphy, the Fat Man shares survival skills in an insane world. He teaches interns to "buff" charts and to "turf" hopeless cases elsewhere (p. 61). He models caring behaviors among patients who can comprehend the care. He invokes 13 laws of the House of God, all raucous and outrageous, but aimed to counterbalance the senseless thrust of an institution to apply technological procedures regardless of human cost. One law reads: "The only good admission is a dead admission" (p. 420). Patients love Fats, and Roy asks, "As crass and as cynical as you are?" (p. 213). Fats answers, "That's why: I'm straight with 'em and I make 'em laugh at themselves. . . . I make them feel like they're still part of life, part of some grand nutty scheme instead of alone with their diseases" (pp. 213–214). Roy reflects on this: "I was touched. Here was what medicine could be: human to human. Like all our battered dreams" (pp. 215–216).

The Fat Man sees his residency as only a part of the nutty scheme of things. He attends to other satisfying occupations. He dabbles with inventions such as his "anal mirror" (p. 107). Fats expounds on his invention: "The anus is a great curiosity to almost all mankind" (p. 107). Roy is never quite sure how tongue-in-cheek this invention idea really is. But the idea reflects a comic relief, a reprieve from the daily grind. Fats models a life outside the House of God. He manages a private practice out of his home, saying, "What's the sense of being a licensed doc if you don't use it 'to relieve pain and suffering'? This GP work is terrific—these are my neighbors, my people" (p. 372). His life connects beyond his occupation at the dehumanizing House of God. Fats touches others; he can also be touched. When an intern commits suicide, Roy recalls that "the Fat Man was crying. Quiet tears filled his eyes, fat wet tears of desperation and loss" (p. 313). Fats can touch Roy: When he comes to apologize for the recent distance between them, he links pinkies with Roy. Roy remembers, "It was perfect, a magical moment. . . . He'd sensed my emptiness, and he'd responded. His touch meant I wasn't alone. He and I were connected" (p. 373).

Fats also helps the interns consider meaningful occupational connections. Toward the end of their rotation, he works with the interns to select specialty areas. Using chalk and a blackboard, he lists the advantages and disadvantages that the interns see in each specialty. The exercise, one largely of values clarification, helps Roy. He says, "By the end of the Fat Man's colloquium, the remarkable had happened: on paper, Psychiatry was the clear winner" (p. 381). Fats is able to touch the lives of the interns. Through caring gestures he helps connect them with meaningful occupations.

Conclusion

Reflection about the art of occupational therapy is less widespread in the professional literature than is reflection about the science of occupational therapy. This is a matter of concern in that occupational therapy is a blend of art and science. The art of practice includes the ability to establish rapport, to empathize, and to facilitate choices about occupational and human potential within a community of others. Engaging in the art of practice commits the therapist to an encounter with an individual who is a collaborator in his or her plan for treatment. Collaboration includes a discussion of each patient's personal goals and of professional and personal assumptions about both the human condition and the meaning of occupation in a life. Without the caring elements that ground the therapist–patient relationship and the dialogue that grounds collaborative treatment planning, occupational therapy would be reduced to a sterile science of occupation.

The current health care system does not encourage the art of practice. Medical practitioners, propelled by the scientific model, have recently returned to a consideration of their lost art. Systematized patient defenses against the depersonalization and fragmentation of their care have affirmed the popular need for care in addition to cure. Practitioners looking to sustain their art have had to turn to sources other than the health care system. The new discipline of literature and medicine attempts to support a humane medical practice through the insightful reading of fiction, and it has the potential to sustain the art of occupational therapy practice as well. By reading fictional literature in its fullest, aesthetic sense, one can reflect on and affirm the importance of relationships and caring in practice by comparing and contrasting those various personal characteristics most conducive to helping. Reading fictional literature in its moral sense can enable practitioners to explore values and assumptions about the human condition and, more specifically, about the importance and meaning of occupation in a life. This reading process is adaptable to the educational system as well as to any other continued education format.

Examples from three fictional works illustrate that both positive and negative images of occupational therapy and occupation can affirm commitment to artful practice. Reading fiction can validate the competence, mastery, and human connectedness with others possible through occupation. Reading fictionalized stories of occupational therapists and other caregivers can affirm those personal qualities of warmth, genuineness, humor, and empathy that are essential in the establishment of a helpful bond.

The art of occupational therapy practice requires validation, though perhaps not in the same manner as does its science. The reading of fictional literature can provide occupational therapists with sustaining images: images of relationships, images of qualities that make relationships meaningful, and images of the meaning of occupation in a life. Reflection on these images can reaffirm one's commitment to the art of providing occupation as therapy.

Acknowledgments

I extend special thanks to Dr. Anne Hudson Jones, Institute for the Medical Humanities, The University of Texas Medical Branch, whose flexibility and encouragement made it possible to integrate course material with occupational therapy issues. I also thank Doreen S. McCarty for typing the manuscript.

References

American Occupational Therapy Association Council on Standards. (1972). Occupational therapy: Its definition and functions. *American Journal of Occupational Therapy, 26,* 204–205.

American Occupational Therapy Association Representative Assembly minutes—1981. (1981). *American Journal of Occupational Therapy, 35,* 792–802.

Coles, R. (1979). Medical ethics and living a life. *New England Journal of Medicine, 301,* 444–446.

Devereaux, E. B. (1984). Occupational therapy's challenge: The caring relationship. *American Journal of Occupational Therapy, 38,* 791–798.

Engel, G. L. (1977). The need for a new medical model: A challenge for biomedicine. *Science, 196,* 129–135.

Jones, A. H. (1987). Reflections, projections, and the future of literature-and-medicine. In D. Wear, M. Kohn, & S. Stocker (Eds.), *Literature and medicine: A claim for a dis-cipline* (pp. 29–40). McLean, VA: Society for Health and Human Values.

Kesey, K. (1962). *One flew over the cuckoo's nest.* New York: New American Library, Signet Books.

Mosey, A. C. (1981). *Occupational therapy: Configuration of a profession.* New York: Raven Press.

Pellegrino, E. D. (1979). In M. J. Vogel, & C. E. Rosenberg (Eds.), *The therapeutic revolution: Essays in the social history of American medicine* (pp. 245–266). Philadelphia: University of Pennsylvania Press.

Rebeta-Burditt, J. (1977). *The cracker factory.* New York: Bantam Books.

Reed, K. L., & Sanderson, S. R. (1983). *Concepts of occupational therapy.* Baltimore: Williams & Wilkins.

Shem, S. (1978). *The House of God.* New York: Dell Publishing.

Trautmann, J. (1978). The wonders of literature in medical education. In D. Self (Ed.), *The role of the humanities in medical education* (pp. 32–44). Norfolk, VA: Teagle & Little.

Yerxa, E., & Sharrott, G. (1986). Liberal arts: The foundation for occupational therapy education. *American Journal of Occupational Therapy, 40,* 153–159.

The Depersonalization of Patients: A Profile Gleaned from Narratives

Suzanne M. Peloquin

Key Words: professional–patient relations • therapeutic use of self

Occupational therapists who would better understand and advocate against depersonalization in health care can find specific references in narratives to the attitudes and behaviors that seem problematic. Patients argue that helpers fail to recognize that illness and disability are events charged with personal meaning. Instead of communicating with patients, helpers establish a distance that diminishes them. They withhold information in a manner that precludes hope, they use brusque manners, and they misuse their powers. Each of these behaviors seems unreasonable and impersonal, and each discourages patients. Together these narratives might inspire therapists to value interactive reasoning as central to practice, to recommit to their consideration of persons, and to enact a climate of caring.

Suzanne M. Peloquin, PhD, OTR, is Associate Professor of Occupational Therapy, School of Allied Health Sciences, J-28, 11th and Mechanic Street, University of Texas Medical Branch at Galveston, Galveston, Texas 77555–1028.

This article was accepted for publication April 20, 1993.

Patients say that their experiences with health care practitioners are difficult, describing their grasp of the problem with the words *dehumanizing* or *depersonalizing*. The abstractions have become the shorthand expression for a dismay that persons who seek health care are often treated carelessly. But what do depersonalizing behaviors look like? Woven throughout a large number of narratives is a profile of impersonal attitudes and behaviors that patients say discourage them when they most need courage. Such a profile can be a powerful resource for therapists who aim to truly care for patients.

More than a decade ago, several therapists addressed the concept of caring at the 60th Annual Conference of the American Occupational Therapy Association in Denver, Colorado (Baum, 1980; Gilfoyle, 1980; King, 1980; Yerxa, 1980). Their collective message encouraged practitioners to recommit to caring, continue the profession's tradition of arguing the dignity of persons, and shape the social climates within which they practice. Yerxa (1980) further argued that occupational therapists can become powerful advocates for a climate of caring because of their unique perspectives.

This article summarizes one step in a larger inquiry into the climate of caring. Conducted between January 1990 and September 1991, the inquiry researched the following as they relate to the encounters that patients have with caregivers: (a) personal narratives that describe impersonal treatment; (b) the historical events and societal constructs that have shaped the patient–helper relationship; (c) empathy and the manner in which helpers learn to be empathic; (d) the nature, practice, and experience of art; and (e) the proposition that empathy might be cultivated through the use of art. Each step of the inquiry required an extensive literature review in each of the areas specified: phenomenological narratives, the social sciences, history, philosophy, and the arts. From each review a number of major themes emerged, and these were subjected to reflection, analysis, and synthesis.

The literature that describes unhelpful encounters between patients and their helpers is the subject of this article. This literature review includes stories about the experience of illness and disability because encounters with caregivers often appear in these. Articles from behavioral science and health professional journals published within the last 10 years also served as resources when their titles suggested some consideration of the patient–helper relationship. Of more than 100 vignettes found, those included in this article most clearly delineate the unhelpful behaviors and attitudes of helpers and clarify the meaning of depersonalization in a compelling manner.

Sarason (1985), a clinician who is troubled by the carelessness of helpers, identified one reason for any caregiver to listen to a number of stories:

> In a vague, inchoate way, people feel and know that the clinical endeavor has become problematic, that those who are in helping roles are both cause and victim, that something is wrong somewhere, and that, far from getting better, it seems to be getting worse. (pp. 203–204)

The personal hurts described in narratives may hone a vague feeling that something is wrong into a keener understanding.

Other reasons for occupational therapists to consider such stories can be found in the literature that emerged during the same time period as this investigation. Within the context of clinical reasoning, Fleming (1991) asked therapists to consider face-to-face interactions with patients as the "interactive" or "underground" practice that often goes unreported (p. 1011). Her observations of the clinicians who participated in the clinical reasoning study suggest that therapists do not always articulate the interactional aspects of their behaviors as central to practice:

> It seems that although the therapists did not initially recognize interaction and interactive reasoning as central to their practice, they used it at least as an adjunct to practice on many occasions for various reasons. (p. 1010)

But this underground practice was important to patients, and the narratives included in this discussion affirm its importance. When patients' encounters with helpers fail to communicate the attempt to understand that is the hallmark of interactive reasoning, treatment will not be felt as therapy (Fleming, 1991). Armed with the clarity and specificity of complaint that the narratives in this selection depict, occupational therapists might more clearly perceive and openly affirm interactive reasoning as a central part of their treatments.

The concept of caring for and interacting with patients as persons is not new to the profession. Arguments that the patient–therapist relationship matters have been variously articulated within discussions of moral treatment (Bing, 1981; Peloquin, 1989a), the therapeutic use of self (Frank, 1958; Peloquin, 1990), and the art of practice (Devereaux, 1984; Mosey, 1981; Peloquin, 1989b). But there is much merit to arguing that these concepts are central to the reasoning process. Embedding the patient–therapist relationship within *clinical reasoning* might allow therapists to reconceptualize caring as a reasonable activity as opposed to a merely expressive adjunct. Providing occupational therapists with compelling stories that illustrate the effects of uncaring attitudes and behaviors might inspire them to care. Together, the reconceptualization and the inspiration might empower therapists to create a day-to-day climate of caring.

The Narratives

Within the body of literature on clinical reasoning, Mattingly (1991) suggested that "perhaps occupational therapy as a profession needs to take its phenomenological tasks more seriously" because the phenomenological perspective is "neglected as an articulating and legitimizing framework for practice" (p. 986). Phenomenological narratives that speak to the nature and consequences of impersonal treatments need to be taken seriously. Patients say that practitioners act in a way that belies any claim to understanding. Patients say that because of a new and special connection that illness spins, practitioners become significant others but do not seem to recognize their heightened significance.

Patients say that helpers depersonalize health care practice by failing to see the personal consequences of illness and disability. They deny the feelings of those whom they treat; they ignore patients and dismiss their concerns. They fail to show, even in small ways, that they are persons who feel, who participate in their patients' pain. Instead they engage in distancing behaviors and harmful withholdings; they are silent, aloof, and brusque. They misuse their power. Patients say that these behaviors discourage them when they are in much need of encouragement. Stories such as these can serve as a legitimizing framework for promoting the kinds of actions that encourage.

Eric Hodgins, a former editor of *Fortune* magazine, spoke to those assembled at a meeting of the American Association for the Advancement of Science in 1964. His address later graced the *Annals of the New York Academy of Sciences* as a well-crafted essay about his medical treatment after a stroke. Because Hodgins's experience happened at mid-century and is the earliest story included in this discussion, his comments lead each wave of patient complaints about the various actions that depersonalize.

Failure to See the Personal Consequences of Illness or Disability

Hodgins (1964) has regretted that practitioners fail to recognize illness as an experience of personal problems.

> If the patient's personality, his trade or job, and the residual disabilities with which his stroke has left him — if these factors line up adversely enough, then a depressed and perhaps despairing human being has now supplanted, in February, someone who, in January, was earning his living, supporting his family, and planning the events of his own future. In my own case, I found it both depressing and infuriating that I encountered no physician with the willingness or capacity to say, "Yes, I agree you are in a jam — in fact several jams." (p. 839)

Hodgins wanted his caregivers to understand that his cerebrovascular accident had damaged far more than his brain. His stroke meant much more. For example, Hodgins had lost considerable dexterity, and, because he could no longer button his shirt, he imagined that he could no longer appear in public, let alone return to work. Although he squeezed a manual gauge with a growing strength that pleased his physician, he had lost the fine capacity to compose at his typewriter—the essence of his passion, his livelihood, and his connection with others. Hodgins's treatment neglected these "jams" of his illness; no one supposed his grief, sense of incompetence, or loneliness. He wanted solutions to his physical problems, but more than these, he sought someone who grasped their deeper meaning in his life. He needed to hear a practitioner say "I understand what this must mean to you, and I am so sorry about your losses." Instead, surrounded by practitioners who attended to his bodily functions, Hodgins faced the meaning of his stroke alone.

Benziger (1969) struggled with the emotional jams of her chronic depression: "I must accept the fact that my illness may recur . . . I must accept the fact that fear does and will jump out at me at the most unexpected moments, and haunt me for no apparent reason" (p. 166). She grieved most when her fear careened between herself and others, but she believed that illness prompted her heightened sensitivity: "An abrupt word, or a harsh one, can bring resentment, anger, and a desire to retaliate" (p. 166). Beisser (1989) agreed that illness is an emotional prod:

> Overwhelming feelings greatly sensitized me to those who cared for me. I scrutinized the countenance of my attendants for their every mood and whim. Everything that affected them affected me. If I was cared for willingly and without reluctance, I felt good and the world was sunny. If my care was given grudgingly or irritably, in a callous way, powerful feelings of degradation swept over me. (p. 33)

In this manner, anger joins fear, and their companionship in illness is not surprising. Murphy (1987) felt the anger, often stifling his "hoarse and futile cry of rage against fortune" (p. 106) against an ill-fated force that made a stranger of him and a tangle of his relationships. Beisser (1989) recalled his pain when, pushed by anger and fear to seek some connection with another, he met disregard: "It was lonely, and I longed to be touched. I sometimes thought that I was like a leper or an 'Untouchable'" (p. 25). Patients ask practitioners to be roused by what they feel; they long for their approach. But some helpers cannot fathom their patients' feelings.

Practitioners enlarge the social unease of their patients with unthinkable expectations. Murphy (1987) thus peered out from inside his own paralysis to recognize it as a "disease of social relations" (p. 20). His caregivers assigned him this burdensome task: "Don't complain!" The unspoken demand made of patients is that they smile and be happy. Sacks (1984) rejected the role of the happy patient after his leg injury, angered at being allotted a social status different from that which he normally enjoyed as a neurologist:

> I found I was avoided by the nonpatients in the garden—the students, nurses, visitors who came there . . . .We had been stamped, with the stigmata of patients, the intolerable knowledge of affliction and death, the intolerable knowledge of passivity, lost nerve, and dependence—and the world does not care to be reminded of such things. (pp. 163, 165)

Practitioners let patients join their social relations on condition that they stifle their pain. When patients wear their wounds too openly, they risk transmitting a case of unease. Distance seems the best defense against such contagion. Instead of seeing that patients want helpers to approach them and infer what they must feel, many practitioners recoil from the stigmata and the pain. And any helper who forces patients such as Hodgins (1964) to then wonder who *will* care adds to the burden of illness this question:

> From whom, then, is the patient to draw courage without which he will not truly recover? Not from a silent practitioner, not from a stuffy practitioner; not from a practitioner, whether doctor, therapist or nurse, who is aloof. (p. 841)

One who is silent, stuffy, or aloof answers clearly that patients may not draw courage from practitioners. That answer evokes another wave of complaints about how helpers hold patients at arms' length, or further away. For example, Browne and Freeling (1976) remembered a newly appointed physician who questioned his predecessor about his role, to get this reply: "Oh! It is all quite straight-forward old boy, your job here is purely and simply to keep the patient at bay" (p. 21). And so enjoined, helpers practice many forms of keeping patients at bay, developing expertise in making distance.

The Distance That Dismisses

The distance experienced by Hal Lear was unbreachable (1980). He sat in the office of a psychoanalyst, hoping to quit smoking after his massive heart attack. The doctor started to hypnotize him, as planned, asking him to relax and close his eyes; without warning, Lear caught the change: "It was not the doctor's voice live. It was the doctor on tape, a stereophonic blast repeating the idiot phrases again and again, while the doctor himself might be out having lunch" (p. 84). Absenting himself, this doctor had depersonalized quite literally—without warning, without explanation, and without any sense of what his disappearance might mean to his patient. He treated his presence lightly, his patient impersonally.

Patients expect that practitioners will attend to them and talk to them; when helpers cut these basic connections, they hurt their patients. Because helpers claim to be there, patients expect them to notice what happens; they often fail to do so. For example, one man had his hand broken when a transportation aide accidentally pushed his gurney into a cart (Jacques, 1983). Back in his room and wearing a splint, he remembered that "a nurse helped him into bed, told him his lunch would be there soon, and left saying, 'Have a good day.' He couldn't believe that she hadn't noticed his hand" (p. 18). Her parting words, careless under the circumstances, added the insult of inconsideration to his injury. Surely she *meant* no harm. But a helper who notices selectively causes patients pain. Belknap (Belknap, Blau, & Gross-

832

man, 1975) recalled an instructor who was known as an excellent diagnostician: "He told a young woman that she had multiple sclerosis and that with time her nerves would degenerate . . . .He then moved on to the next case, never seeing the shock and fear in her eyes or the disquiet on the faces of the staff" (p. 14). He never considered what the diagnosis and its consequences meant to this young woman; he failed to grasp her feelings. He did not attend, but stood off from these matters instead.

When patients worry that helpers might not notice, and therefore ask them to attend, they often do not. Beisser (1989) shared the pain and rage that such dismissive care evokes:

> I would call the nurse and ask for another blanket to cover me. The room seemed comfortable to her, so she would doubt my judgment. In order to check, she would usually reach down to feel my leg. Then she would say something like "Oh, it's all right, you're not cold." (pp. 18–19)

How secure practitioners seem with such pronouncements! But how can anyone presume to know better than patients what they feel? It is this senseless inattention to their experience that patients call impersonal.

Narratives about patients who have felt altogether left out of their treatment are almost a cliché. When patients feel excluded, it is because practitioners have treated them lightly. Murphy (1987) told this story:

> One morning in the hospital, a nurse was washing me when she was called away by another nurse who needed help in moving a patient. "I'll be right back," she said as she left, which all hospital denizens know is but a fond hope. She left me lying on my back without a call bell or the TV remote, the door was closed, and she was gone for half an hour. Wondering whether she had forgotten me, I tried to roll onto my side to reach the bell. But I was already quadriplegic, and, try as I might, I couldn't make it . . . .I thought then of Kafka's giant bug, as it rocked from side to side, wiggling its useless legs, trying to get off its back—and I understood the story for the first time. (p. 108)

And consider another pointed story in which a nurse's aide described her patient as a 96-year-old woman immobilized after a stroke (L.E.P., 1987). The aide's task was to get the patient out of bed, and she outlined her plan to an assistant: "I'll take an arm and a leg on this side, you take an arm and a leg on that side and then . . . ." Her words were interrupted by the alert and personable patient: "Oh, God, she's not even going to make a wish!" (p. 53). It is as if practitioners somehow believe that as they tend to their problems, patients are not there. And when patients press practitioners to see that they *are* still there, many hold them at bay.

Harmful Withholdings

Hodgins (1964) suggested that when helpers' dismissals consist of silences, patients feel these as withholdings: "I am thinking of the enigmatic smile after the blood pressure readings and the utter silence after examining retinal blood vessels . . . .I am thinking of the nurse's stolid mask

after removal of the thermometer from wherever it was" (p. 841).

Hodgins was bright and curious, but he did not believe that he was singular in wanting to learn the reason for or the results of a procedure done in his presence. He felt that knowing his condition would allow him to better understand and take part in his treatment. Utter silence angered him. His anger seems legitimate; when patients seek information, helpers' withholdings create new problems for them. Caregivers withheld much from Leete (1987):

> I resent the fact that I was not given information about my illness and the methods used to treat it, some of which I feel were harmful. For example, alternating electroshock with insulin coma therapy in 1966 only served to virtually eradicate my memories while probably adversely affecting my ability to learn new information. Doing so without my awareness was criminal. (p. 486)

Most patients argue that they have a reasonable stake in the outcome of their treatments. When practitioners give silent treatments that both dismiss and deprive them, patients wonder why any helper might so readily discount a patient's interest in care. Lear repeatedly asked about his condition because he wanted to know what to expect (1980). His persistent inquiries led many of his practitioners to tag him a "bad patient"; he was often denied information. After he found the severity of his problems through a solitary investigation of his records, his anger erupted: "*None* of you understood; *the truth would have been easier*" (p. 267). Only with some clarity about what he might expect did Lear feel that he could muster the courage to face his illness.

Discouraging Words

Often when practitioners break silence to share more than an enigmatic smile, they fail to fathom that it may be comfort or hope that patients seek. They furnish discouraging words rather than helpful information. Hodgins (1964) explained whose courage such words seem to muster:

> It seems to this patient that many persons in medicine today continue to foster and cherish mystery for mystery's sake. I am thinking of the prescriptions still written illegibly in pig Latin . . . .I am thinking of what H. W. Fowler called love-of-the-long-word . . . .All such conventions exist for the convenience and protection of doctors; their effect and *perhaps* their intent is to diminish the patient. (p. 841)

Even when helpers use technical terms not so much to diminish their patients but to hand them the truth, Lee (1987) wrote that they forget the ferocity found in their words:

> A hematologist examined me. He had a closet of pet lions, and his recommendations unleashed several for my contemplation. Their mouths were open. "Although she is still clinically, [*sic*] in Stage III, the severity of the symptoms makes more widespread involvement a possibility. Because of this, chemotherapy (MOP) is in order" . . . .These lions stayed in my room. At times they were very big, and I would tremble. Sometimes they were small, but they were always present, with teeth. (p. 110)

Many practitioners are blind to the fears that they unleash. Because medical language is so familiar to them, they choose their words without care. It then sometimes surprises them that even simple words hold different meanings for their patients. A medical student explained, "Last week someone quoted the example of a woman who was told she had a tumor and she responded with, 'Oh well, I'm glad I haven't got cancer.'" (Moore, 1978, p. 165). Too often, patients say that the concerns and words of practitioners differ from their own. Patients want to know how they might face their illness, but helpers think in other terms.

Practitioners, according to Coles (1989), are taught to think in abstractions, such as "a phobic, a depressive, an acting-out disorder" (p. 17). These terms work against their understanding the meaning of these illnesses to their patients; the labels remove helpers from the reality that the patient's experience is one of fear, sadness, or anger. Coles remembered how William Carlos Williams fretted about the pervasive use of abstractions in health care:

> I can say, "The patient is phobic" — not a callous or coldhearted or impersonal attitude, but a brief, pointed piece of information shared with another busy professional. Yes; but Dr. Williams had this amplification: "Who's against shorthand? No one I know. Who wants to be shortchanged? No one I know." (p. 29)

Helpers often shortchange patients. Instead of speaking everyday language that might let patients share their sense of the illness or let helpers tell their own concern, they choose words that camouflage meaning. They hold conversations impersonally, lest they catch their patients' pain. Instead of saying "I know that you are frightened" and risking a portion of that fear, they announce "You have a phobia" and remain unaffected. Helpers cherish words that discourage patients.

Brusque Behaviors

Sometimes it is not so much meaningless or dispassionate long words that discourage patients as it is ill-considered remarks. Hodgins (1964) regretted the brusqueness, the negligence of good manners, the disregard for the bedside manner:

> Its connotations used to be straight; now they are crooked. To say that a physician had a good bedside manner was once to say that he brought hope and comfort to his recumbent or expiring patient; now the phrase is more likely to be a sneering jibe. (p. 843)

Courtesy and social graces are increasingly uncommon in health care practice. Benziger (1969) remembered, "A rather cross-looking old woman came into my room and locked my clothes closet, my bureau, and my bathroom. 'But I have to use the bathroom during the night,' I protested. 'That's your problem,' she said" (p. 34). Brice (1987) recalled an equally upsetting event. After surgery for an ileostomy, she suffered an excruciating pain that she thought signified a bowel obstruction. She sent her husband out to beg the nurses to help, because, up until that point, she had failed to convince them that she had pain. She remembers that a charge nurse soon "barrelled" into the room, saying "I want you to quit moaning and quit manipulating" (p. 31). When the nurse returned a few minutes later to see on the floor the 1000 ccs of vomitus that confirmed the obstruction and the pain, she said "Oh shit!" but nothing else.

Even worse is this story. Jacques (1983), a patient representative, soothed a patient who had naively asked the doctor if her neck brace might have caused her problems. She told Jacques,

> "He flew into a rage and called me a 'smart ass'!" When she tried to explain, the doctor told her that he didn't like his patients telling him what to do, told her that she could get another doctor, and then discharged her. (p. 106)

When practitioners behave so brusquely, patients cannot possibly sense that their enlarged sensitivity or fragile courage is understood.

There is also this piece that appeared in a medical journal (Nicky, 1982). An older woman emerged from a taxi in the winter of 1981, "cold, feeble, and wobbly on her feet." She was confused by the crowds and by the din of the clinic where she met brusqueness head-on:

> Behind a "cage" a few feet away she saw a young and pretty clerk. As the elderly lady, full of hope, approached the counter, a sharp voice stopped her: "Stay in line." Which line? she pondered. She felt incapable of either arguing or waiting. First nausea, headache, blurry vision, fever, unsteady gait. Now this! She broke into tears. Why did she venture to get help? She went home to die. . . . A neighbor found her *in extremis* and called an ambulance. She was dead on arrival at the hospital. (p. 1906)

The consequence of keeping this woman at bay was fatal. Although an illustration, perhaps, of ill-considered remarks in the extreme, the story underscores the power of practitioners: People may die if helpers do not care. This story also differs from that of Hodgins, Murphy, or Sacks because it is told by another, one who is not a patient. Many patients like this woman, who never take pen in hand to protest, are often those who feel dismissal in the form of prejudice. An old woman with yellowed hair and failed hearing may not get an explanation because she is judged incomprehending. A black man wearing tattered clothes may wait for hours because his time is judged less valuable. An unkempt teenager who reeks of liquor might face rough handling because her life is judged loathsome. Patients like these hear sharp demands to "stay in line" because they are seen as having stepped beyond some value-laden boundaries set up by their practitioners. Although genuinely ill, these patients attract labels like *difficult* or *noncompliant* that rationalize the hidden bias of their helpers while mitigating their care. Prejudice moves the story of this man, judged both ignorant and hostile:

> The gunshot victim is brought into the trauma unit of the hospital with very unstable vital signs. The doctors and nurses immediately set about stabilizing the patient. One of the nurses starts an IV in

834

his left arm, while an intern calls for a Foley catheter tray so he can insert the catheter . . . .While the intern inserts the catheter, a resident decides to do a rectal examination. Naturally, the patient reacts to the probing finger.

> Doctor: Damnit, RELAX!
> Patient: Hey man, be cool. Just ask nice. You don't have to cuss me out, just ask nice and you don't have to jab your finger up my ass.
> Doctor: Shut up. And relax. We know what we're doing.

The patient seems to be stabilizing because the vital signs are improving . . . .It is at this point that the senior surgical resident decides to put down an NG tube.

> Doctor: Hey man, just cool it. Relax, this isn't going to hurt.
> Patient: Doc, look, I've had one of those things before and it wouldn't go in my nose. They had to put it into my mouth.

The doctor struggles to insert the tube.

> Doctor: Damnit, stay still, I'm trying to save your life!
> Patient: Hey doc, I appreciate that, but man, I'm scared and I know you can't put that tube in my nose. Other doctors have tried and they couldn't. They had to put it in my mouth.
> Doctor: Look, tie him down so I can get this tube in. I'm not going to fool around all night with this guy. (Holderby & McNulty, 1982, pp. 91–92)

The doctor did not fool around much longer. The patient had a cardiac arrest while trying to get loose. Two nurses who later protested were reported as unprofessional.

Many health care narratives show helpers grappling with their powers. There is, of course, the awesome power that illness holds over the balance of a life—whether and how it might be lived. But life-changing power also dwells in treatments. Patients seek some position from which they might control these powers and their fears. Hodgins, for example, yearned to hear a practitioner say, "You will encounter some difficulties no one can foresee, but for most of these *you will find your own individualistic solutions*. It will take time, but it will happen" (p. 840). With these words, he might have taken heart. But instead of hearing words that might turn him toward his own resources, Hodgins felt locked out of his care and powerless.

The Misuse of Power

The next wave of patient complaints protests a mismanagement of power:

> Almost everyone who has been in a hospital has seen examples —perhaps not in his own case—where neglect of this truism [that the patient is part of his treatment] has brought the relationships between patient and health personnel to the point of being adversary proceedings. (Hodgins, 1964, p. 842)

Hodgins believed that it is reasonable for an ill person to fret over what might happen next. Given the despair that often stalks illness, a patient's wrestling control of steps along the course of treatment is understandable. Equally understandable is another patient's frantic abandonment of choice to someone thought in a better place to fix the problem. When ill with cancer, Harris (Harris & Stripling, 1980) shared what must be every patient's unspoken fear over whether to take or yield control:

> When am I going to be able to control my life and be able to make my own decisions? I realize the doctors know what is best for me

medically, but do they know what is best for me mentally as well? Doctors need to realize that I'm not just a patient number, a tumor, or a disease, but that I am a human who needs a sense of security, a feeling of responsibility, a feeling of control over what is happening in my life and what I think should be done about it. (p. 20)

But in battles for command over what will happen, the patient depends on the practitioner and often withers in conflicts over choosing. Brice (1987) remembered the one-downmanship:

> When, with the naivete of a layman, my husband asked him why I wasn't getting better, my surgeon twice-protested that he was sure it wasn't *his* fault. Thinking he might take offense, my husband and I were frightened of being forthright in requesting a second opinion. At that point my care was too critical. My life hung too precariously in his hands. (p. 31)

If helpers could imagine how frightened and troubled patients are, they might expect them to seek other opinions and curse mistakes. But all too often practitioners interpret patient challenges as personal assaults rather than reasonable expressions of distress. When practitioners admit that much outstrips their knowledge or control, patients can be quite forgiving. Martha Lear (1980) remembered a medical student who tried to draw blood from her husband. The young man explained that he was nervous. He apologized profusely after his third failure to angle the needle correctly. Hal Lear appraised the student favorably: "That kid was nervous, but he wasn't a snot . . . . He was concerned. You can learn to give an injection, but you can't learn concern. He'll be okay" (p. 218). Lear's pessimism about whether concern can be learned is sad. But stories in which practitioners elbow into or out of patient rooms, conversations, and lives justify such pessimism.

Conclusion

The voices within these narratives send out a steady plea. The central complaint is that when practitioners depersonalize, they are not inclined to care, and their behaviors sap a patient's courage. Helpers rarely listen when patients ask them to attend; patients then reason that practitioners lack the required sensitivity. They despair of being understood.

When helpers neglect their patients' heightened sensitivity, they intensify the pain of illness. At a time in their lives when patients need someone to be there, helpers hold them at bay. They press patients, who experience little control and much anxiety, to be good. They ask for compliance even as they become evasive, curt, or arrogant. They then seem startled to stir a patient's anger; they are baffled when a struggle ensues.

Practitioners withhold important information as part of taking charge. They fail to talk about the experience of illness, about possibilities, about the future. They rarely broach feelings. They have a hard time saying that they are sorry—for the illness, for the pain, for their mistakes. They have a harder time showing, even in small ways, that they are persons who see, who reflect, and who participate in their patients' pain. They dread that pain.

Helpers sometimes argue that patients long for a magical cure, for the impossible. And at these times they sound like this young physician (Kleinman, 1988):

> There is only so much you can tolerate—all the problems, the calls, all the patients and families. . . . They want so much, every one of them. If this keeps up, I'll either burn out in another year or two or become a danger to my patients and myself" (p. 214)

Because of this threat, many rehearse their distance as students. Helpers might recall, with Coles (1989), this lesson: "I learned it was best for me to be 'cautious, polite, meticulous'; best for me to set aside therapeutic zeal; best for me not to get 'too involved'" (p. 9). And all too often, practitioners set themselves aside; practice becomes impersonal. Helpers feel torn between contradictory pleas that they be sensitive on the one hand and competent on the other. Many don the professional mask only to discover it is of small use when "after midnight, the professional protection is gone. You feel very alone, vulnerable" (Kleinman, 1988, p. 216). Masked, they stay unseen, unknown, guarding against their pain. But, over time, persistence in wearing the mask will stifle them. Slaby (1986), a physician, explained:

> You are not sharing human experiences . . . .The sharing that I have done with my families has sustained me. The sharing relationship with my patients leads to feelings of growing both in wisdom and emotionally as a human being. It actually prevents burnout. (Slaby & Glickman, p. 162)

Although most distancing behaviors aim to safeguard helpers against pain, the distance often thwarts their being unified selves. Practitioners must see that they can step into their patients' worlds with compassion. Any small part of the pain that helpers share makes room in which patients can then turn to their own courage. When practitioners doubt the capacities of persons to encourage one another, they diminish themselves and their patients, forgetting that personal presence is the fundament of care.

Occupational therapists who seek in patients' stories a profile of unhelpful attitudes and behaviors can find them. Anyone who is tempted to see such stories as unlike occupational therapy practice and thus irrelevant might remember the stories told by Parham (1987) or Peloquin (1990) about patient–therapist encounters that were not helpful, such as this one:

> June Kailes, a leader in the Independent Living Movement and Director of the Westside Independent Living Center in Santa Monica, California, is a talented and intelligent woman who happens to have cerebral palsy. Her recollection of therapy is that she was asked repeatedly to drill on tasks like putting beads in jars, presumably for coordination: "Anybody could see that wasn't going to be my thing!" Why had no one attempted to help her channel her considerable intellectual abilities toward more satisfying goals? (Parham, 1987, p. 556)

Those who do not see such practices within their occupational therapy clinics might recall the plea for patient advocacy articulated more than a decade ago by leaders in the profession (Baum et al., 1980). Occupational therapists are part of the larger health care system, and they often work in close proximity to manifestations of the disregard, distance, and impersonality that preclude a climate of caring. Historically, therapists have acted in response to societal trends. Clinicians and educators alike have prepared for the trend to see practice as an accountable business by improving documentation and assuring quality care. They prepare now to meet the needs of tomorrow's large population of elderly patients. It seems at least equally important to carefully consider and advocate against any trend that darkens the countenance of caring.

At the very least, occupational therapists can take from these stories a renewed conviction that the exchanges that patients have with their helpers matter very much. Stories such as these suggest that the time has come to openly support the practice of striving to understand patients as unique persons. One group of therapists speaks to the aptness of doing so: "With the emphasis we have always placed on the person, we have much we can share with others as we try to incorporate a holistic perspective on achieving and maintaining wellness, particularly in the face of adversity" (Hamlin, Loukas, Froehlich, & MacRae, 1992, p. 969). ▲

Acknowledgment

The research for this article constitutes a portion of a dissertation that partially fulfilled requirements for a doctoral degree conferred by the Institute for the Medical Humanities, the University of Medical Branch, Galveston, Texas. The dissertation is entitled *Art in practice: When art becomes caring.*

References

Baum, C. M. (1980). Eleanor Clarke Slagle lecture—Occupational therapists put care in the health system. *American Journal of Occupational Therapy, 34,* 505–516.

Beisser, A. (1989). *Flying without wings: Personal reflections on becoming disabled.* New York: Doubleday.

Belknap, M. M., Blau, R. A., & Grossman, R. N. (1975). *Case studies and methods in humanistic medical care: Some preliminary findings.* San Francisco: Institute for the Study of Humanistic Medicine.

Benziger, B. F. (1969). *The prison of my mind.* New York: Walker.

Bing, R. K. (1981). Eleanor Clarke Slagle lectureship 1981—Occupational therapy revisited: A paraphrastic journey. *American Journal of Occupational Therapy, 35,* 499–518.

Brice, J. (1987). Empathy lost. *Harvard Medical, 60,* 28–32.

Browne, K., & Freeling, P. (1976). *The doctor–patient relationship.* New York: Churchill Livingstone.

Coles, R. (1989). *The call of stories: Teaching and the moral imagination.* Boston: Houghton Mifflin.

Devereaux, E. B. (1984). Occupational therapy's challenge: The caring relationship. *American Journal of Occupational Therapy, 38,* 791–798.

Fleming, M. H. (1991). The therapist with the three-track mind. *American Journal of Occupational Therapy, 45,* 1007–1014.

Frank, J. D. (1958). The therapeutic use of self. *American Journal of Occupational Therapy, 12,* 215–255.

Gilfoyle, E. M. (1980). Caring: A philosophy for practice. *American Journal of Occupational Therapy, 34,* 517–521.

Hamlin, R. B., Loukas, K. M., Froehlich, J., & MacRae, N. (1992). Nationally Speaking—Feminism: An inclusive perspective. *American Journal of Occupational Therapy, 46,* 967–969.

Harris, B., & Stripling, S. (1980). The patient on the receiving end, out of control. *Cancer Bulletin, 32*(1), 20–21.

Hodgins, E. (1964). Whatever became of the healing art? *Annals of the New York Academy of Sciences, 164,* 838–846.

Holderby, R. A., & McNulty, E. G. (1982). *Treating and caring: A human approach to care.* Reston, VA: Reston Publishing.

Jacques, F. (1983). *Verdict pending: A patient representative's intervention.* California: Capistrano.

King, L. J. (1980). Creative caring. *American Journal of Occupational Therapy, 34,* 522–528. Kleinman, A. (1988). The illness narratives: Suffering, healing, and the human condition. New York: Basic.

Kleinman, A. (1988). *The illness narratives: Suffering, healing, and the human condition.* New York: Basic.

Lear, M. (1980). *Heartsounds.* New York: Simon & Schuster.

Lee, L. (1987). Transcendence. In M. Saxton & F. Howe (Eds.), *With wings: An anthology of literature by and about women with disabilities* (pp. 109–116). New York: Feminist Press.

Leete, E. (1987). The treatment of schizophrenia: A pa-tient's perspective. *Hospital and Community Psychiatry, 38,* 486–491.

L. E. P. (1987, July). *Reader's Digest,* p. 53.

Mattingly, C. (1991). The narrative nature of clinical reasoning. *American Journal of Occupational Therapy, 45,* 998–1005.

Moore, A. R. (1978). *The missing medical text: Humane patient care.* Melbourne, Australia: Melbourne University Press.

Mosey, A. C. (1981). *Occupational therapy: Configuration of a profession.* New York: Raven.

Murphy, R. F. (1987). *The body silent.* New York: Henry Holt.

Nicky. (1982). A visit to a renovated clinic. *Journal of the American Medical Association, 127,* 154–157.

Parham, D. (1987). Nationally Speaking—Toward professionalism: The reflective therapist. *American Journal of Occupational Therapy, 41,* 555–561.

Peloquin, S. M. (1989a). Looking Back—Moral treatment: Contexts considered. *American Journal of Occupational Therapy, 43,* 537–544.

Peloquin, S. M. (1989b). Sustaining the art of practice in occupational therapy. *American Journal of Occupational Therapy, 43,* 219–226.

Peloquin, S. M. (1990). The patient–therapist relationship in occupational therapy: Understanding visions and images. *American Journal of Occupational Therapy, 44,* 13–21.

Sacks, O. (1984). *A leg to stand on.* New York: Harper & Row.

Sarason, S. B. (1985). *Caring and compassion in clinical practice.* San Francisco: Jossey-Bass. Slaby, A., & Glickman, A.S. (1986). Adaptation of physicians to managing life-threatening illness. *Integrative Psychiatry, 4,* 162–165.

Slaby, A., & Glickman, A. S. (1986). Adaptation of physicians to managing life-threatening illness. *Integrative Psychiatry, 4,* 162–165.

Yerxa, E. J. (1980). Occupational therapy's role in creating a future climate of caring. *American Journal of Occupational Therapy, 34,* 529–534.

Brief or New

Using the Arts To Enhance Confluent Learning

Suzanne M. Peloquin

Key Words: curriculum • education • students

Suzanne M. Peloquin, PhD, OTR, is Associate Professor, Department of Occupational Therapy, School of Allied Health Sciences, The University of Texas Medical Branch at Galveston, 301 University Boulevard, Galveston, Texas 77555–1028.

This article was accepted for publication March 20, 1995.

An approach named "confluent education" two decades ago by Brown (1971) can enhance the efforts of educators and students to (a) develop understanding of human occupation and human experiences, (b) generate an ease and familiarity with the process of interactive reasoning, and (c) cultivate an empathic attitude. Brown described the approach as follows:

> Confluent education is the term for the integration or flowing together of the affective and cognitive elements in individual or group learning. It describes a philosophy and a process of teaching and learning in which the affective domain and the cognitive domain flow together, like two streams merging into one river. (p. i)

Occupational therapy educators can use the arts as part of confluent education, thereby awakening the affective element of learning that can occur through the mediacy of sensory experiences, metaphors, and imaginative excursions into the lives of others.

The aims of this article are to (a) illustrate the manner in which the visual and literary arts have been successfully integrated, over the past 5 years, into select courses in one undergraduate program and (b) provide a list of resources for interested educators (see Suggested Readings at end of article). Although the academic arena is the specific focus of this discussion, the principle of confluent education generalizes readily to educational efforts during fieldwork or professional development among more seasoned practitioners.

A Rationale for Confluent Education

Confluent education has strong resonance with occupational therapy practice, which is traditionally characterized as a science and an art (American Occupational Therapy Association [AOTA], 1972). A fundamental reason for confluent learning in occupational therapy derives from the belief that the best of practice builds on competence and caring, two excellences that have been identified in the occupational therapy literature (Peloquin, 1990). The image of a competent and caring therapist is that of a thinking–feeling person who engages in both the art and the science of helping others through occupation.

The argument for educational approaches that promote confluence builds on the character of occupational therapy as both cognitive and affective and on the guidelines for educating professionals (AOTA, 1991). Students who ready themselves for any humanistic practice must learn to understand—that is, to think about *and* feel themselves into—the experiences of others. Education that leads students to think and feel promises such understanding.

The arts are a suitable resource for confluent education because they convey both the cognitive and affective meanings that people attach to their lives, their occupations, and their worlds (Peloquin, 1989). Combs, Avila, and Purkey (1971) described the powerful learning that derives from the literary arts:

> Through drama, poetry, autobiography, and novels, it is possible to expand our experience vicariously. We can enter the world of seeing, and feeling, believing, hoping, trusting, caring, loving, and hating in more or less degrees as those experienced by other people. As we give ourselves up to the spell woven by these kinds of writers, we can be for a time what we are not, ever have been, or perhaps never could be. (p. 199)

A similar enriching process, says Gilmour (1986), is true of visual works: "We learn from the pictures we have encountered, and they remind us of the richness of the world" (p. 22). Students can learn much from the human truths and emotions that inspire poems, paintings, plays, or films.

One last practical reason for embracing confluent education is that students respond positively to the approach. Use of the arts has consistently produced comments such as this one: "This instructor's method of teaching is unique and more effective than traditional methods. You can feel the person behind the disorder, the person behind the therapist" (Anonymous, personal communication, 1993).

Applications of the Confluent Approach

The confluent approach makes sense for occupational therapy education. Academic courses can include objectives for emotional, reflective, and sensitive learning alongside more cognitive goals. Brown (1971) supported the implementation of confluent education by minimizing its difficulty:

> What is proposed here is common sense, is something we've known about for some time, is possible within the present educational establishment.... The change would simply be to be aware that thinking is accompanied by feeling and vice versa and to begin to take advantage of the fact. (p. 3)

Brown's (1971) assertion seems valid; art has integrated well into courses as varied as Basic Concepts in Occupational Therapy, an introductory lecture and laboratory course; Interpersonal Practice, an elective laboratory course; and Applied Neurosciences in Occupational Therapy, an intermediate lecture course.

Most classroom sessions that structure these three courses allow several engagements with art as participants move from cognitive to affective considerations. The following activities flow nicely into more traditional lectures and laboratory experiences: reading literary works aloud, showing visual works, and assigning drawing tasks. Although these choices have reflected the personal prefer-

ence of one instructor and a goodness of fit with course objectives, other artful engagements, such as listening to music or performing segments of plays, seem equally apt.

The examples that follow aim to illustrate confluent education: (a) reading a poem to enhance a discussion of human occupation, (b) engaging students in drawing tasks to elicit reflection about the process of helping, (c) showing a visual work of art to exemplify active listening, and (d) reading from fiction and autobiography to increase understanding of neurological conditions and empathy for those who experience them.

Reading a Poem

Within the course entitled Basic Concepts in Occupational Therapy, much discussion targets the constructs of purposefulness and occupation. The following poem, an excerpt from the work of Petersen (1976), adds to this discussion:

> There is a shouting SPIRIT
> deep inside me:
> TAKE CLAY, it cries,
> TAKE PEN AND INK,
> TAKE FLOUR AND WATER,
> TAKE A SCRUB BRUSH,
> TAKE A YELLOW CRAYON,
> TAKE ANOTHER'S HAND–
> AND WITH ALL THESE
> SAY YOU,
> SAY LOVING.
> So much of who I am
> is subtly spoken
> in my making. (p. 61)

Although it takes less than a minute to read, the poem moves conversation toward increased personal reflection and expression of feelings—about what constitutes meaningful occupation, about individual differences, about personal identification with various forms of doing, and about self-expression. The poem's artistry evokes an awareness of the power and the humanizing potential of occupation that rational discourse does not.

Drawing

Drawing is also used in Basic Concepts of Occupational Therapy to teach about helping, collaboration, and the therapeutic use of self—all aspects of interactive reasoning. A drawing task clarifies the thoughts of students as they summarize their grasp of the assigned readings. The instructor draws two circles on the blackboard, naming one *therapist* and the other *patient/client* while asking, "What should I do to this drawing to illustrate a collaborative relationship?" The ensuing discussion is generally a lively mix of suggestions and countersuggestions. Often a student tells the instructor to move the circles closer to one another. Acknowledging this directive, the instructor seeks feedback about how much closer the circles should be. Some students argue for touching circles, others do not. The task uncovers controversial aspects of helping (such as proximity, self-disclosure, and touching) magnified through the drawn image.

Another activity is the instructor's request that students draw constructs and then compare one another's productions. During the Interpersonal Practice course and within a discussion on limit setting and negotiation, students are given the following situation, partly written and partly drawn on the blackboard: Person A wants an equilateral triangle, and Person B wants a circle. Students are asked to draw as many compromises as they can imagine and in so doing to think about their understanding of the term *compromise*. Time spent comparing individual drawings yields various meanings of and feelings about compromise made more specific by this question: "How might the compromise you drew occur with patients or colleagues in the clinic?"

Viewing Visual Art

The painting *Burned Face* by Appel (Janson, 1986) adds feeling to a discussion of active listening during the Interpersonal Practice course. Completed in 1961 in a form of abstract expressionism, the picture is marked by bold colors and vigorous brush strokes. Added to these are daubs and squiggles of orange and flesh. The pigments look thick in places and often crawl and zigzag into one another. Because the work is so abstract it is an apt object lesson in listening past the surface of things.

Students look at either a slide or a reproduction of *Burned Face* as they listen to a 4-minute reflective commentary reproduced in part here:

If one has such a burn, does looking in the mirror or glancing in a store-window cause real doubt about whether one has a face at all? Ugly seams and lumpy blotches replace the once-familiar freckle, the curve and color of lip, the chicken-pox scar, all landmarks that spoke quietly but reassuringly of a once-familiar self. Gone forever are the old ways of pursing the lips, of wrinkling the brow, of closing the eyes.

I am forced to ask whether a face is something I have, or an essential component of who I am. Surely my face is who I am. Without a face to reflect my feelings, could I make my meanings known to others? Without a face, could I ask others to meet and return my gaze? Might I wonder if somewhere under all of this burned flesh my face and I lived on the same as before only trapped behind this hideous mask? Or might I understand that I had in some awful moment turned into ropey flesh? I would lose a large measure of what I know to be me if I were to lose my face tomorrow. And so it must be for a

patient so burned. (Peloquin, 1991, pp. 281–282)

After this experience, when students are asked, "What are the risks of really listening?" and, "What are the risks of not listening?" they share both their thoughts and feelings.

Reading Literary Works

A final example of using the arts as part of confluent education is the reading of excerpts from fiction or autobiography during each of the 15 lectures of a course entitled Applied Neurosciences in Occupational Therapy. Whether the topic is homonymous hemianopsia or coma, Parkinsonism or schizophrenia, some personal story about what the condition or the treatment *feels* like finds equal footing alongside relevant neurological considerations. The inclusion is easy; it seems natural to share the meaning of these disorders, and students attend to the stories with palpable interest.

Conclusion

Confluent education is consonant with the nature of persons and congruent with the character of occupational therapy. Integrating the visual and literary arts within a variety of courses is one viable application of the construct. Confluent learning, with its integration of thought and feeling, offers the hope of developing competent practitioners who also care. Such learning also holds promise for developing the kind of understanding described by Stevens and Rogers (1976):

There are two ways to ride a horse (or drive a car, or clean a house, or take care of a garden, or teach, or build, or anything else). One rider demands that the horse be o[b]edient to him, he makes the horse a "thing." If he has any feeling for the horse it is the feeling of possession, of "mastery." The other kind of rider is, with his horse, more like a centaur—horse and rider move together, responding to each other in a way that makes them move as one; they understand each other. (pp. 130-131) ▲

References

American Occupational Therapy Association. (1972). Occupational therapy: Its definition and functions. *American Journal of Occupational Therapy, 26,* 204–205.

American Occupational Therapy Association. (1991). *Essentials and guidelines for an accredited educational program for the occupational therapist.* Rockville, MD: American Occupational Therapy Association.

Brown, G. I. (1971). *Human teaching for human learning.* New York: Viking.

Combs, A. W., Avila, D. L., & Purkey, W. (1971). *Helping relationships: Basic concepts for the helping profession.* Newton, MA: Allyn & Bacon.

Gilmour, J. (1986). *Picturing the world.* Albany: State University of New York Press.

Janson, H. W. (1986). *History of art.* Englewood, NJ: Prentice Hall.

Peloquin, S. M. (1989). Sustaining the art of practice in occupational therapy. *American Journal of Occupational Therapy, 43,* 219–226.

Peloquin, S. M. (1990). The patient–therapist relationship in occupational therapy: Understanding visions and images. *American Journal of Occupational Therapy, 44,* 13–21.

Peloquin, S. M. (1991). *Art in practice: When art becomes caring.* Unpublished doctoral dissertation, University of Texas Medical Branch at Galveston, Texas.

Petersen, J. (1976). *A book of yes.* Niles, IL: Argus.

Stevens, B., & Rogers, C. (1976). *Person to person: The problem of being human.* Lafayette, CA: Real People Press.

Suggested Readings

The Visual Arts

Aries, P. (1985). *Images of man and death.* Cambridge, MA: Harvard University Press.

Berg, G. (1983). *The visual arts and medical education.* Carbondale, IL: Southern Illinois University Press.

Coln, R. N. (1969). *Medicine in art.* Minneapolis: Lerner.

Death and the visual arts. (1977). New York: Arno Press.

Gerdts, W. H. (1981). *The art of healing: Medicine and science in American art.* Birmingham, AL: Birmingham Museum of Art.

Gilman, S. (1982). *Seeing the insane.* New York: Brunner/Mazel.

Gilman, S. (1988). *Disease and representation: Images of illness from madness to AIDS.* Ithaca, NY: Cornell University Press.

Janson, H. W. (1991). *History of art.* Englewood Cliffs, NJ: Prentice Hall.

Jones, A. H. (Ed.). (1988). *Images of nurses: Perspectives from history, art, and literature.* Philadelphia: University of Pennsylvania.

Jung, C. G. (1966). *The spirit in man, art, and literature.* New York: Pantheon Books.

Karp, D. R. (Ed.). (1985). *Ars medica.* Philadelphia: Philadelphia Museum of Art.

Kiell, N. (1965). *Psychiatry and psychology in the visual arts and aesthetics.* Madison, WI: University of Wisconsin Press.

Naumburg, M. (1950). *Schizophrenic art.* New York: Grune & Stratton.

Pringhorn, H. (1972). *Artistry of the mentally ill.* New York: Springer-Verlag.

Reitman, L. (1951). *Psychotic art.* New York: International Universities Press.

Richardson, B. E. (1969). *Old age among the Greeks.* New York: Ams Press.

Rooselot, J. (1966). *Medicine in art.* New York: McGraw-Hill.

Selzer, R. (1928). *Mortal lessons: Notes on the art of surgery.* New York: Simon & Schuster.

Three hundred years of American painting. (1957). New York: Time, Inc.

Literary Arts

Brody, H. (1987). *Stories of sickness.* New Haven, CT: Yale University Press.

Carmichael, A. G., & Ratzon, R. M. (Eds.). (1991). *Medicine: A treasury of art and literature.* New York: Hugh Lauter and Levin Associates.

Ceccio, J. (1978). *Medicine in literature.* White Plains, NY: Longman.

Coles, R. (1989). *The call of stories: Teaching and the moral imagination.* Boston: Houghton Mifflin.

Feder, L. (1980). *Madness in literature.* Princeton, NJ: Princeton University Press.

Gubler, D. V. (1971). *A story of illness and death in the lives and representative works of Leo Tolstoy and Thomas Mann.* Provo, UT: Brigham Young University.

Hillman, J. (1983). *Healing fiction.* New York: Talman Co.

Hughes, J. M. (1969). *The dialectic of death in Poe, Dickinson, Emerson, and Whitman.* Philadelphia: University of Pennsylvania.

Jung, C. G. (1966). *The spirit in man, art, and literature.* New York: Pantheon Books.

Kleinman, A. K. (1988). *The illness narratives.* New York: Basic.

Kranfeld, D. A. (1978). *The mad character in modern literature.* Providence, RI: Brown University.

Mersand, J. E. (1961). *Three plays about doctors.* New York: Washington Square Press.

Mukand, J. (Ed.). (1990). *Vital lines: Contemporary fiction about medicine.* New York: St. Martin's.

Self, P. (1984). *Physical disability: An annotated literature guide.* New York: Decker.

Silverberg, R. (1974). *Drug themes in science fiction.* Rockville, MD: National Institute on Drug Abuse.

Tesser, S. O. (1957). *Fiction and the unconscious.* Boston: Beacon Press.

Trautmann, J. (1975). *Literature and medicine: Topics, titles, and notes.* Philadelphia: Society for Health and Human Values.

Trautmann, J. (Ed.). (1981). *Healing arts in dialogue: Medicine and literature.* Carbondale, IL: Southern Illinois University Press.

Trautmann, J. (1982). *Literature and medicine: An annotated bibliography.* Pittsburgh: University of Pittsburgh Press.

Zola, I. K. (Ed.). (1982). *Ordinary lives: Voices of disability and disease.* Cambridge, MD: Apple-Wood Books.

The Fullness of Empathy: Reflections and Illustrations

Suzanne M. Peloquin

Key Words: history • professional–patient relations

Seven core values are said to undergird the profession of occupational therapy, with empathy serving as a hallmark of one of those values — personal dignity. This inquiry explores the meaning of empathy within a practice that holds occupation at its center. The literature on empathy in both philosophy and the behavioral sciences yields cogent thoughts about the fullness of empathy and its characteristic actions. The Healing Heart, *the biography of a pioneer therapist, Ora Ruggles, shows the manner in which occupational therapists can be empathic in their practice. These reflections and illustrations serve to sharpen the vision of occupational therapists as persons who reach for both* the hands *and* the hearts *of others.*

Suzanne M. Peloquin, PhD, OTR, is Associate Professor, Department of Occupational Therapy, School of Allied Health Sciences, The University of Texas Medical Branch at Galveston, 301 University Boulevard, Galveston, Texas 77550-1028.

This article was accepted for publication April 14, 1994.

The American Occupational Therapy Association (AOTA, 1993) has identified seven core values that undergird the profession: altruism, equality, freedom, justice, dignity, truth, and prudence. These values "provide a basis for clarifying expectations between the recipient and the provider of services" (p. 1086). The document on core values can also be seen as part of an effort to shape and secure a vision of practice. For therapists who work in a range of settings with distinct frames of reference, a clear vision promises a clear identity, a shared purpose, and a source of inspiration. The title *occupational therapist* keeps occupation at the center of the vision; the profession's enfranchisement of common values can hone the character of its practice.

According to AOTA's identification of core values, a therapist honors personal dignity through an "attitude of empathy" (AOTA, 1993, p. 1086). The words are familiar, but their meaning must be clear if occupational therapists are to develop this attitude. What does empathy *look* like? More pointedly, what does it mean to be empathic in a practice that holds occupation at its center?

This discussion explores these questions, moving from thoughts on the full-bodied nature and actions of empathy to illustrations of the empathic practice of a pioneer therapist. The literature on empathy in both philosophy and the behavioral sciences structures this inquiry. Several ideas articulated by artists, caregivers, and philosophers who have been associated with the topic appear verbatim because their power to evoke reflection is remarkable. Time spent with well-spoken ideas and clearly rendered images sharpen one's sense of what it *means* to be empathic. Because this inquiry occurred simultaneously with the research done on clinical reasoning (Fleming, 1991; Mattingly, 1991), the conclusions that emerge from this work can be said to resonate with and support that effort rather than derive from it.

The Nature of Empathy

Saint Exupéry (1971/1943) argued in *The Little Prince* that many persons relinquish their capacity to imagine and to feel, attending instead to grown-up matters:

> I showed my masterpiece to the grown-ups, and asked them whether the drawing frightened them. But they answered "Frighten? Why should anyone be frightened by a hat?" My drawing was not a picture of a hat. It was a picture of a boa constrictor digesting an elephant. But since the grown-ups were not able to understand it, I made another drawing: I drew the inside of the boa constrictor, so that grown-ups could see it clearly. They always need to have things explained. . . . The grown-ups' response this time was to advise me to lay aside my drawings of boa constrictors, whether from the inside or the outside, and devote myself instead to geography, history, arithmetic and grammar. That is why, at the age of six, I gave up what might have been a magnificent career as a painter. (p. 4)

Similar experiences pull many persons away from their involvement with imagination and feeling. Devoting themselves to other matters, they lose sight of their power to see beyond the surface of things. But when the 6-year-old in this story grew into an adult, he often used his childhood drawing to predict the quality of understanding that he could expect from others. He explained:

> I have lived a great deal among grown-ups. I have seen them intimately, close at hand. And that hasn't much improved my opinion of them. Whenever I met one of them who seemed to me at all clear-sighted, I tried the experiment of showing him my Drawing Number One, which I have always kept. I would try to find out so, if this was a person of true understanding. But, whoever it was, he, or she, would always say: "That is a hat." Then I would never talk to that person about boa constrictors, or primeval forests, or stars. I would bring myself down to his level. I would talk to him about bridge, and golf, and politics, and neckties. And the grown-up would be greatly pleased to have met such a sensible man. (p. 5)

It is not only in fanciful stories like Saint Exupéry's that one finds references to both the innateness and the frequent relinquishment of the capacity to understand. Katz (1963) shared a similar belief:

> A simple way to explain the origin of the empathic skill is to postulate that we are born to understand. Part of our biological heritage is the capacity to visualize and to apprehend the feelings of other members of our species. We do not locate this ability in a particular sense organ. It is simply a function of our inner senses, an imaginative or intuitive gift which is part of human nature. (p. 62)

Katz argued that children often surrender to a more detached use of imagination and intuition because in Western culture parents and teachers favor objective and logical responses.

One who would have a voice and place in any health care practice must be sensible, but one who would also be empathic must retain the capacity to apprehend, imagine, and feel. Helpers must convey understanding as they strive to solve health care problems. As Leder (1984) said, "One must look at a human not just as body but as body *and* mind" (p. 38). Bruner (1986) reminded practitioners that, as with the stereoscope, depth is better achieved by looking from two points at once; the dual perspective to which Bruner referred evokes the nature of empathy. Reed (1984) explained its structure of opposites:

> First, there are the active and passive versions of the clinical experience of empathy—the former associated with grasping meaning, understanding, and interpreting; the latter with resonating, sudden illumination, losing the self. Second, there are the rational and mystical sides to the concept of empathy—the first associated with concepts such as perceptual scanning, organization of derivatives, and inference; the second, usually rejected, with telepathy and the uncanny. Third, there is the opposition between science and art, in which the dispassionate observation of data that leads to uncontaminated understanding contrasts with the creative resynthesis of data. (p. 16)

Not surprisingly, Katz named empathy's supposed mystical quality problematic in Western culture because it suggests a somewhat "divinatory art" (p. 11).

The dichotomous aspects of empathy no doubt relate to the dual origins of the word in the psychology of aesthetics and in the psychology of understanding other persons (Olinick, 1984). In 1897, Lipps, as noted by Katz (1963), introduced the term *einfuhlung* into his writings on aesthetics to explain how a person "feels into" an art object to appreciate it:

> An observer is stimulated by the sight of an object and responds by imitating the object. The process is automatic and swift, and soon the observer feels himself into the object, loses consciousness of himself, and experiences the object as if his own identity had disappeared and he had become the object himself. The observer sees a mountain and apprehends it with his inner imaginative activity, his muscles as well as his eyes. As his gaze moves upward to the peak of the mountain, his own neck muscles tense and for the moment there is the sensation of rising. He is not aware of the sensation, however. He experiences the mountain not as a static object of great height but as an object which extends and rises from the valley to the clouds. (pp. 85–86)

In the scheme proposed by Lipps, one enters into art objects, apprehending them in terms of some personal experience. One sees a container and projects into it the human act of holding. One apprehends a tree swaying or a leaf falling as a person might; one personifies. When persons understand a work or art in terms of what happens to them in the world, they engage in empathic appreciation.

Interpersonal meanings became associated with the word *empathy* later, when Titchener (1909) described the act of reading the movements of another as a rendering of einfuhlung. But such a term need not have had two points of origin to lay claim to its complexity. The duality of reasoning and feeling that constitutes empathic understanding reflects the rational-emotional constitution of persons. The problem is that empathy's structure of opposites has made the concept prey to the one-sided regard for reason that prevails in Western culture. The dilemma experienced by patients as depersonalization seems one of an imbalance and disharmony in favor of rationality (Peloquin, 1993). The problem reflects an impoverishment of empathy.

Helpers need a way of knowing persons and their illnesses that transcends the linear approach and prepares them to treat *persons*. Hayakawa (1969) described the tenuousness of any one way of knowing:

> The thermometer, which speaks one kind of limited language, knows nothing of weight. If only temperature matters and weight does not, what the thermometer "says" is adequate. But if weight, or color, or odor, or factors other than temperature matter, then those factors that the thermometer cannot speak about are the teeth of the trap. Every language, like the language of the thermometer, leaves work undone for other languages to do. (p. 8)

The language of health care practitioners has warranted scrutiny because it seems cold and uncaring; it is a knowing that seems inadequate. Practitioners need fluency in the discourse about pain and courage, and that discourse requires the capacity to think and feel at once.

The Actions of Empathy

Those who remember material learned from courses or textbooks may want to dismiss any discussion of empathy because of those associations, thinking, "Oh, another rehash of how to decode body language and paraphrase what the patient says." Any such dismissal would be hasty, because such thinking disregards the essential actions of empathy. Katz articulated the challenge: "Being human," he said, "means more than being a physicochemical unit. To be a man means to be a fellow man. The human personality becomes human through its association with others" (1963, p. 189). Association with others is a function that persons should not relinquish lightly. Instead, asked Perlman (1979), "Might not even a specialist be more 'human'? Might not even a 'skin man' say, be taught to reconnect with the human self he was before he immersed himself in becoming a professional expert, so as to relate to the patient who is a person *under* the skin?" (p. 7)

How can practitioners relate to their patients as fellows? Thomas (1983b) explained that such a relationship rests first on their willingness to present themselves:

> My host was the newly elected president of the society, a general practitioner in his fifties, a successful physician whose career was to be capped that evening after the banquet, by his inauguration; to be president of the county medical society was a major honor in that part of the world. During the dinner he was called to the telephone and came back to the head table a few minutes later to apologize; he had an emergency call to make. The dinner progressed, the ceremony of his induction as president was conducted awkwardly in his absence, I made my speech, the evening ended, and just as people were going out the door he reappeared, looking harassed and tired. I asked him what the call had been. It was an old woman, he said, a patient he'd looked after for years; early that evening she had died, that was the telephone call. He knew the family was in distress and needed him, he said, so he had to go. (p. 10)

The disposition to be there that is central to empathy is also fundamental to Buber's (1965) concept of dialogue, in which one person turns toward the other, "of course with the body, but also in requisite measure with the soul" (p. 10). The turning in dialogue is an empathic action, and it demands more than rational procedures; it asks more of who one is than of what one does. Empathy seems to be the heart of what practitioners mean when they profess to attend to their patients. Likening it to love, Hackney (1978) saw empathy as a qualitative response to persons, a potential possessed.

Adler (1931) believed that if practitioners did attend to patients more fully, they would see a kinship: "To understand is to understand as we expect that everybody should understand. It is to connect ourselves in a common meaning with other people, to be controlled by the common sense of all mankind" (p. 254).

Empathy spins connections through which helpers *see* their own likeness to their patients, in eyes that widen, brows that furrow, hands that clench. But empathy also quickens a respect for differences. At its deepest level, Egan (1986) explained, empathy is a way of seeing with the eyes of others to appreciate nuances in their visions of the world. To be present for one's patients empathically is to take a stand from which one partici-

pates in their experiences. Such a supportive stance is aptly named an understanding.

Perhaps the description of empathy that is most cited in the behavioral sciences is that offered by Rogers (1975), who depicted a person enacting this "strong yet subtle and gentle" response:

> It means entering the private world of the other and becoming thoroughly at home in it. It involves being sensitive, moment to moment, to the changing felt meanings which flow in this other person, to the fear or rage or tenderness or confusion or whatever, that he/she is experiencing. It means temporarily living in his/her life, moving about in it delicately without making judgments. . . . as you look with fresh and unfrightened eyes at elements of which the individual is fearful. . . . In some sense it means that you lay aside your self and this can only be done by a person who is secure enough in himself that he knows he will not get lost in what may turn out to be the strange and bizarre world of the other. (p. 3)

In his early writings, Rogers (1957) underscored the as-if cognition that sustains the empathic response: one thinks and feels and moves as if one were in the patient's world. This imaginative presence enables practitioners to clearly differentiate their patients' experiences and feelings as separate from, if like, their own. If practitioners aim to help, Reiser and Schroder (1980) explained that they must know how to be there for their patients, fiercely caring, while standing as themselves — the hallmark of empathy:

> Having been on both sides, I have developed a strong conviction that doctors who are practicing effectively cannot, and should not, become so welded to their patients psychologically that they feel no difference between their patients' pain and their own. In order to help people who are sick, we must know what it is like to be in their shoes but, at the same time, also know very well that we are not in their shoes. (p. 46)

Practitioners sometimes seem ambivalent about intimacy. They worry that "they may not be able to extricate themselves from the net of feeling" (Katz, 1963, p. 25). When they stand overwhelmed with feelings, however, it is not empathy that they enact, but sympathy. Olinick found sympathy "an immature, imperfect empathy" (1984, p. 139). Sympathetic helpers never quite get out of themselves; they touch the patient's feelings and duck back into their own worlds, grasping only the certainty that they hurt, too. But the empathizer, said Katz, "tends to abandon his self-consciousness" (p. 9). And even if a helper engages in a profound act of empathy, "the power to recover" remains (Katz, p. 42).

Empathy does not exact a fusion but a connection. It implies an experience not only of the pain of another, but of the integrity and courage that dwell alongside the pain. Empathy, in health care practice, is the enactment of the conviction that, empowered by someone's willingness to understand, the patient will gather the requisite measure of courage.

The empathic way of being asks that practitioners feel and think at once. In embracing their own feelings, practitioners reclaim themselves. The potential for such reclamation is great; the universality of the capacity was argued by Thomas (1983a) on the occasion of his visit to the Tucson Zoo:

> I was transfixed. As I now recall it, there was only one sensation in my head: pure elation mixed with amazement at such perfection. Swept off my feet, I floated from one side to the other, swiveling my brain, staring astounded at the beavers, then at the otters. . . . It lasted, I regret to say, for only a few minutes, and then I was back in the late twentieth century, reductionist as ever. (p. 8)

Thomas (1983a) took from his experience the conclusion that the unalterable patterns of response, ready to be released in persons by such encounters, is one of affection.

Practitioners who would understand their patients must be similarly disposed. Every person can find a wealth of happenings to awaken or reawaken human affection. For some it may be the sight of frolicking otters, for others the sound of a river rushing or the scent of newly mown grass. For occupational therapists, the story of the empathic practice of a pioneer therapist might occasion such a reawakening.

The Healing Heart: The Story

The story of Ora Ruggles (Carlova & Ruggles, 1946) chronicles much of the early history and professionalization efforts of occupational therapy from World War I through the 1950s. With a strength of character honed by childhood events, Ruggles responded to the wartime call for crafts experts to "reconstruct" disabled soldiers. Assigned first to Fort McPherson, Georgia, as a reconstruction aide, Ruggles marshalled supporters and supplies despite bureaucratic blocks. She engaged ever larger groups of soldiers in craft work that reduced their restlessness and restored meaning to their lives. She quickly engaged the interest and the emotions of each patient in order to make her efforts therapeutic.

Her accomplishments gained acknowledgement from Army administration and physicians alike. Patients responded to her competence, warmth, and concern with a mixture of awe, loyalty, and thanks. After a romantic involvement with a patient who died, Ruggles left the fort, emotionally devastated.

Eleanor Clarke Slagle, one of the founders of the National Society for the Promotion of Occupational Therapy, pressed her to return to Army work. Ruggles did, establishing occupational therapy departments among patients with tuberculosis in Tucson, Arizona, and in California, at both the Santa Monica Sanatorium and the Sawtelle Soldier's Home. Her employers saw her success as a type of magic, but her approach assumed a recognizable pattern.

She changed her patients' environments, engaging them in that process to increase their interest and optimism. She researched local techniques and supplies. She earned trust and forged warm bonds while showing

patients what occupational therapy could do. She overcame cynicism. She adapted activities and fashioned ways in which even persons with severe disabilities could succeed.

After her discharge from the Army in 1927, Ruggles established a number of occupational therapy departments in California, and one in Kula, Hawaii, on the island of Maui. Her departure from Hawaii coincided with the bombing of Pearl Harbor. While at Olive View, a sanatorium in the San Fernando Valley, Ruggles faced personal exhaustion and emotional impoverishment. Her career had filled her life; she had lost the concept of achieving a balance in work, play, and self-care. Ruggles took a year off for worldwide travel and then trained others to meet the need for wartime therapists while she ran a shop to sell crafts made by patients.

Ruggles, now revitalized, resumed work at Children's Hospital in Los Angeles, starting an occupational therapy department in typical pioneer fashion. After being abruptly hospitalized for appendicitis, Ruggles ended up in a psychiatric ward due to an allergic drug reaction that produced symptoms of restlessness and agitation; her caregivers unwittingly continued to give her the drug that threatened her life. Responding to an uneasy sense that Ruggles might need help, a minister friend called a nurse, and the two went to the hospital to find Ruggles in an isolation room. They saw to it that the wrongful medication was discontinued. This frightful event renewed Ruggles' zeal for humane hospital work. She continued at Children's Hospital, welcoming the challenge of younger patients, but being deeply affected by their struggles and deaths.

After a number of years, Ruggles retired and faced great difficulty with her new role. An occupational therapist friend reminded her to use the principles of occupational therapy in her own case. Remembering the principle of activity as a healing agent, Ruggles launched into a full life of painting, volunteering in her community, and helping other retirees.

The Healing Heart, though perhaps romanticized, gives a view of early practice within an accurate historical context. Because the story deals openly with the values that Ruggles held and the relationships that she shared, it lends itself well as an object lesson in empathy.

Illustrations of the Fullness of Empathy

Because the manner of *being with* in occupational therapy is a unique enactment of *doing with*, portrayals of that enactment are important to the vision of practice. In its fullness, empathy calls for a disposition that is active and grasping but also passively receptive; a presence that is concurrently rational and emotional, an act of analytical observation balanced against one of holistic synthesis. Occupational therapy practitioners who would be empathic must reflect the duality of thinking and feeling in their disposition, presence, and actions.

One affirmation of the fullness of empathy lies in the title *The Healing Heart*, derived from a comment made twice by Ruggles, once at the beginning of the story and again at the end. On the first occasion, Ruggles went into the army barracks at Fort McPherson unusually quiet. Her friends noted her mood. They asked whether she was in trouble again with the command. She said that she had made a great discovery, one that she could not get over because it was so simple, yet so effective. When pressed to share, Ruggles said: "Just this. It is not enough to give a patient something to do with his hands. You must reach for the heart as well as the hands. It's the heart that really does the healing" (Carlova & Ruggles, 1946, p. 69). On her retirement from Children's Hospital, when asked by a reporter from the *Los Angeles Times* what the most important element of her work was, she repeated her discovery. A life's work had affirmed her early vision: A patient held both hands and heart within the grasp of one who would reach for them. The fullness of this vision of the thinking-feeling powers of patients shaped Ruggles' practice of empathy.

Ruggles believed the thinking-feeling capacities of therapists to be as important as those of her patients. When she hired helpers, she chose them "not only for their technical skill as therapists but for their warmth and enthusiasm as human beings" (Carlova & Ruggles, 1946, p. 174). She embodied skill and warmth in her exchanges. She was held in awe by patients like this soldier who saw the risks in feeling:

> Everybody needs help, and the fighters in life need it more than anyone else. Courage and strength are not enough. Sensitivity and understanding are necessary, too. It's the sensitive fighters like you, Ma'am, those who aspire to a victory beyond the physical boundaries of their own particular war, who have the capacity for real tragedy. (p. 45)

One instance of Ruggles' use of basket weaving shows the thinking and feeling disposition, presence, and actions that characterized her practice as empathic. At Fort McPherson, Ruggles worked among soldiers who had had amputations secondary to war injuries. She worked two enormous wards, the scenes of much horse-play among those who could hobble, much stone-faced staring from those who could not. A tall and attractive redhead, Ruggles drew much attention on the day she first walked the wards. One patient named Hap, who had no legs and one arm, made Ruggles laugh with his flirtatious comments and impish grin. When she announced that she would keep the men occupied with basket weaving, Hap quipped that he'd rather keep *her* occupied. Another patient, Kilgore, called Hap a legless clown, not man enough to keep anyone occupied. The men grew silent. Ruggles moved to Hap's side and put her hand on his shoulder, saying, "Don't mind him, Hap! Man is far more than an arm or leg" (p. 57). Her words went deep. Within minutes, more than 20 men clamored to get into

her class. Hap later confided that Kilgore was far worse off because he carried a much deeper wound in his "crippled soul" (p. 60).

Because of his disability, Hap could only pass reeds to the other men in the class, and Ruggles felt his new silence as his incapacity became clear. She spent much time thinking about what Hap could do to gain the benefits of reconstruction. She went to the artificial limb shop where limb-making was still rather crude. She described and sketched what she wanted: a leather device from which metal braces and a clamp would protrude. She later approached Hap, cautioning him against too much hope as she slipped the leather breeching over his stump and secured a slender brush within the clamp. As Hap painted tentative lines of colored dye onto the rim of a basket, he whooped with joy. He practiced secretly for days before showing his skill. The men responded with delight; even Kilgore was impressed. Overwhelmed with feeling, Ruggles began a practice that she kept for years. She slipped away from the group into a closet and let the tears flow. That closet was the first of Ruggles' many "crying corners" (p. 63).

Kilgore worried Ruggles. During one class a soldier jeered that Kilgore did not try basket weaving because he knew he could not succeed. Challenged, Kilgore sat for an hour weaving furiously with his huge hands. When one soldier said that the result was not bad, Kilgore drove his fist down to destroy the basket. Ruggles asked the physician about Kilgore's behavior. The physician told her that Kilgore had been a cowboy and that wartime revulsion filled him with anger. Ruggles consulted the foreman of the blacksmith shop and then looked for Kilgore. When she found him and he told her not to ask him to make more baskets, Ruggles showed him a design for spurs and asked if he would help her start a metalwork class. Within the hour he was in the shop, where he mastered the work readily. His drinking, gambling, and violent outbursts stopped, and after discharge he started an ironwork plant —one that grew to be the largest in the Southwest. Kilgore wrote Ruggles, years later:

> I've been doing a lot of thinking lately, Ruggie. It started out last week when some of the boys around town asked me to run for mayor. It makes me realize, again, Ruggie, how much I owe you. I wonder what the boys who asked me to run for mayor would think if they knew an army doctor once scribbled on my medical record, "This man is a menace to society." (p. 91)

Ruggles' treatment of Hap and Kilgore depicts a therapist whose doing with patients reflects the best of analysis, rationality, and action alongside the finest synthesis, sensitivity, and receptivity. Ruggles' enactment of occupational therapy, her reaching for the heart as well as the hands of others, reveals the fullness of empathy.

The Actions of Empathy

Stories within *The Healing Heart* also reveal the many

actions that constitute empathy. The empathic encounter has been said to consist of the following aspects: (a) an expression of *being there*, (b) a turning of the soul, (c) a recognition of both likeness and uniqueness, (d) an entry into the other's experience, (e) a connection with the other's feelings, (f) a power to recover from that connection, and (g) a personal enrichment that derives from these actions. Each of these aspects can be expected to assume a unique character in occupational therapy, in which a therapist brings to the encounter not just the self, but the trappings of occupation: objects, tools, and activities. Although many stories in *The Healing Heart* preclude full consideration of these aspects, select examples illustrate their meaning.

Ruggles was present to her patients in many ways, and one form of her *being there* was the manner in which she helped to reconstruct environments so that her presence and therapy could be extended. One such reconstruction occurred shortly after Ruggles arrived at the Kula Sanatorium. Ruggles was given a stark room with a few tables and chairs. When three patients arrived on her first day, they moved to the windows to be closer, Ruggles thought, to the color and warmth of the world outside. Ruggles quickly got permission to redecorate the workshop. She and her patients made colorful drapes. They painted warm murals of Chinese, Japanese, Hawaiian, and Korean scenes. They made bright cushions for the floor. One elderly woman, much cheered by the room, brought others to chat in the new surroundings, which were much warmer than the wards below. The room had a presence that drew patients to Ruggles and to occupation.

Ruggles' capacity to be there and do with her patients went far beyond creating atmospheres that cheered and supported them. When she worked at Soldier's Home, for example, Ruggles worked with many men who had mental illness, then described as shell shock. One young patient named Mike had driven a truck that overturned, killing six soldiers who had been riding in the back. Mike occasionally ran through the wards in a daze, veering corners as if still driving that truck. Ruggles wondered whether he might benefit from some task that resembled driving. When she consulted the physician, and he asked what that task might be, Ruggles said she needed to think it through. The next day, as she worked with the older patients on a Japanese garden, they struggled to flatten the loose soil with a heavy roller. They jokingly asked if Ruggles knew any heavy men. Minutes later, Mike was moving the roller with deftness and power.

Although Mike continued to have subdued moods, he was much improved. One day as he and Ruggles stood by an army truck, Mike worried aloud about whether he would be ready for discharge. Suddenly he climbed into the truck, set the ignition, and climbed out to crank it. Stunned and frightened, Ruggles raised her voice in pro-

test as Mike clambered back into the cab. Ruggles quickly followed. When he told her to get out because she might not be safe, Ruggles said, "I know I can't stop you, but I'm going along with you" (Carlova & Ruggles, 1946, p. 146). Mike drove well, and when he finished, he slumped against the seat exhausted, musing that nothing lurked in the shadows. He was released a few months later. Clearly, Ruggles demonstrated her commitment to the requisite presence implied in the act of doing with.

Empathy also requires a turning to another that is a *turning of the soul*. One example of Ruggles' turning, not just to solve a problem but to capture and feel its deeper meaning, was her treatment of a child named Ruby at the Children's Hospital. When Ruggles first met Ruby, she saw a most unattractive 12-year-old who retaliated against the taunts of other children by destroying their work. Hoping to explore the child's interests, Ruggles asked Ruby if she might like sewing. The child responded, "Why? So I can grow up and be an old maid and sit at home with my sewing? Is that what you do?" (Carlova & Ruggles, p. 215) Although Ruggles' initial urge was to "whallop" Ruby, she checked her inner heat in remorse and thought, "This girl dislikes people because she can see they dislike her. I must alter my attitude. I must change my hate to love. I must show Ruby that I love her" (Carlova & Ruggles, p. 215). This turn of the soul prompted Ruggles to ask Ruby what she aimed to be when she grew up. In a tiny voice, Ruby said that she hoped to work in a beauty parlor. Ruggles softened as she saw this child in light of her yearning for beauty. She taught Ruby how to shampoo and set her hair, and she arranged for Ruby to spend time in a beauty shop. Over time, Ruggles noticed a change: As Ruby connected with others, her beauty emerged from within. Ruggles' turning of the soul generated a similar turning in her patient.

Another action of empathy is *recognition of likeness* within another, of connecting with the commonality of problems that persons share. Ruggles' work with an 11-year-old boy named Ramon serves as an example of her capacity to understand the need for belonging and to structure occupations to meet that need. Ramon was thought to be incapacitated: He had little voluntary muscular control, and he twitched and jerked constantly. Painfully shy, he hid himself in dark corners so as not to be noticed. One day, when the rest of Ruggles' charges complained that their clay was so lumpy that they were wasting time pressing it through a screen, Ruggles thought of Ramon. She walked him from a corner into the workroom. As soon as he saw the others making clay figures, he reproached Ruggles for suggesting that he join this group. Ruggles countered by showing him how to press clay through the screen. His uncontrolled shaking worked to his advantage, and the other children patted him on the back and thanked him for producing clay with such a fine texture. Ramon felt useful and appreciated, and after a short period he was no longer shy. The task gave Ramon a chance to connect with others in a venture that highlighted fellowship rather than differences.

But empathy also requires a *recognition of uniqueness* in the other, and Ruggles consistently saw differences as challenges to her creativity. Ruggles' practice in a mental ward at Fort McPherson introduced her to some dramatic examples of schizophrenia, during an era before psychotropic medications were developed. One day during her craft class, a patient announced that he was General Pershing and that Ruggles ought to salute. She did. Another patient whispered as they were working that he was a German spy. He and Ruggles agreed on a set of signals they would use to communicate. Ruggles knew another patient to be a bird lover. He stood for hours by the barred windows. One day while he was hallucinating, he demanded to know what the birds were doing in Ruggles' hair. Without pausing, Ruggles said, "Oh those. Their nest was blown away and I'm sort of helping them out until I find another one" (Carlova & Ruggles, 1946, p. 100). Calmed, he complimented the quality of her nest. She learned to salute, to pass secret signals, and to live with the birds as she worked with the men. Her matter-of-fact acceptance of their delusions and hallucinations permitted their engagement with her and with the work that calmed them.

Central to empathy is the act of *entering into the experience of another* to understand what it must be like. Ruggles' interaction with a man named Leo exemplifies her typically sensitive participation in the lives of her patients. Poverty troubled many of the patients at Olive View, especially those with families. Ruggles ran a shop at the sanatorium where patients sold their crafts to allay some of that worry. After Leo arrived he was soon sent to bed with a high fever. He was restless and troubled. He had a wife and four children to support, and his small farm was mortgaged. His family needed $15.25 a month to keep the farm. The physician thought Leo's temperature too high and work with Ruggles too risky. Although Ruggles accepted that decision, as Leo's condition worsened, she reopened the question of his working at a craft. Ruggles thought that Leo's deterioration was more mental than physical. She proposed to work with him at his bedside but to stop if his temperature rose. The physician agreed. Ruggles told Leo that he could make $20 a month selling leather work. Although his first efforts were crude, before long he was producing fine items. His first earnings amounted to $22.65 and the physician's pronouncement that he was well enough to work outside the ward. Leo became Ruggles' leather work assistant, helping other patients as soon as he had made enough to secure his $15.25 a month. Ruggles' work was credited with saving Leo's farm, his pride, and his life. Her willingness to enter into his situation had engaged him.

Ruggles' work among persons who felt so much pain offered many occasions to *connect with their feelings*, another of the actions of empathy. Ruggles helped pa-

tients turn to their courage even when her own feelings were at risk. While Ruggles was on the ward one day, a young soldier who had been shot with shrapnel in 65 places caught her eye as he frantically scanned the room. Kilgore warned her that the young man was about to explode his feelings, and that she'd better go. "They pour it all out at once, then they never talk about it again," Kilgore said (p. 87). Ruggles told Kilgore that she would stay. The soldier spoke of screams in a trench where he sank into a mass of the flesh of his buddies. Suddenly an artillery blast blew him free, and he woke to find parts of bodies, naked, torn, and bloody, scattered all over. "I was the only man alive," he said, "and I wished I was dead" (p. 88). Ruggles sat near the boy for a long time feeling sick and weak. Kilgore whispered that now she too had been through the war, but that she would know better the next time. "No," Ruggles said, "if I can help, I'll stay" (p. 88). As part of their doing with, Ruggles' patients often needed to speak their anguish and share their pain. Ruggles' staying power in the face of their feelings confirmed her empathy.

Her many connections with others led Ruggles to crying corners where she faced the depth of her own feelings:

> Sometimes she felt an almost overwhelming urge to tear herself free and run to the outside world, the world of the well and the normal. Time after time, she resisted the urge, only to feel a more subtle, more agonizing strangulation. The many patients who reached out for her help pained her with the ever increasing pressure of their demands and needs. She stared into the darkness and, assailed by a crushing feeling of futility and helplessness, turned her face to the pillow and wept. (p. 184)

But Ruggles' *power to recover from connection*, another of the actions that is a requisite for empathy, stayed strong. She turned to friends who would listen. She changed jobs to work with different populations. She applied to herself the principles of her therapy, seeking purpose in satisfying forms of occupation. And always, Ruggles saw her practice as one from which she derived the *personal enrichment* that is the promise of empathy. She saw the results of her efforts: through occupational therapy, patients found their own strengths. And Ruggles knew that in "helping others, she helped herself" (p. 191). As the years passed and she felt the growing presence of a supreme spirit, she "felt more than rich" (p. 192).

Summary

Artists, caregivers, and philosophers who reflect on empathy speak to a capacity to understand that builds on the rational-emotional nature of persons. In health care, empathy can be seen as an enactment of the conviction that, empowered by someone's willingness to understand, the patient will gather a requisite measure of courage. Empathy is characterized by an expression of being there, a soul turning, a recognition of likeness and difference, a participation in the experience of another, a connection with feeling, a power to recover from that connection, and a personal enrichment. The disposition, the presence, and the actions of empathy reflect a thinking and a feeling that happen at once.

Empathy assumes a unique character in occupational therapy, a practice in which therapists bring the trappings of occupation to the personal encounter. The story of Ora Ruggles exemplifies both the fullness and the actions of empathy in occupational therapy: a doing with that leads a person to discover inner strength. The picture of empathy found within *The Healing Heart* is that of one person reaching for the hands and heart of another. The picture shows how one can be there while holding occupation at the center of practice; it affirms the belief that an empathic attitude shows deep respect for the dignity of others.

In *The Little Prince* (Saint Exupéry (1971/1943), the pilot recalled his initial reluctance to reach out:

> I did not know what to say to him [the little prince]. I felt awkward and blundering. I did not know how I could reach him, where I could overtake him and go on hand in hand with him once more. It is such a secret place, the land of tears. (p. 31)

But he entered that land and was changed forever; it was an awakening that stirred his heart. Occupational therapists can walk with their patients, reaching for hands and hearts, as did Ruggles, in the land of illness and tears. The enactment of empathy, wherever it occurs, is a reawakening of the heart. ▲

References

Adler, A. (1931). *What life should mean to you.* Boston: Little, Brown.

American Occupational Therapy Association. (1993). Core values and attitudes of occupational therapy practice. *American Journal of Occupational Therapy, 47,* 1085–1086.

Bruner, J. S. (1986). *Actual minds, possible worlds.* Cambridge, MA: Harvard University Press.

Buber, M. (1965). *Between man and man.* New York: Macmillan.

Carlova, J., & Ruggles, O. (1946). *The healing heart.* New York: Julian Messner.

Egan, G. (1986). *The skilled helper: A systematic approach to effective helping.* Monterey: Brooks/Cole.

Fleming, M. H. (1991). The therapist with the three-track mind. *American Journal of Occupational Therapy 45,* 988–996.

Hackney, H. (1978). The evolution of empathy. *Personnel and Guidance Journal, 57,* 35–38.

Hayakawa, S. I. (1969). Introduction. In G. Kepes, *Language of vision* (pp. 1–11). Chicago: Paul Theobald.

Katz, R. L. (1963). *Empathy: Its nature and uses.* London: Free Press of Glencoe.

Leder, D. (1984). Medicine and paradigms of embodiment. *Journal of Medicine and Philosophy, 9*(1), 29–43.

Mattingly, C. (1991). What is clinical reasoning? *American Journal of Occupational Therapy, 45,* 979–986.

Olinick, S. L. (1984). Empathy and sympathy. In J. Lichtenberg, M. Bornstein & D. Silver (Eds.), *Empathy I* (pp. 25–166). New York: Analytic.

Peloquin, S. M. (1993). The depersonalization of patients: A profile gleaned from narratives. *American Journal of Occupational Therapy, 47,* 830–837.

Perlman, H. H. (1979). *Relationship: The heart of helping people.* Chicago: University of Chicago Press.

Reed, G. S. (1984). The antithetical meaning of the term 'empathy' in psychoanalytical discourse. In J. Lichtenberg, M. Bornstein, & D. Silver (Eds.), *Empathy I* (pp. 7–25). New York: Analytic Press.

Reiser, D., & Schroder, A. K. (1980). *Patient interviewing: The human dimension.* Baltimore: Williams & Wilkins.

Rogers, C. R. (1957). The necessary and sufficient conditions of therapeutic personality change. *Journal of Consulting Psychology, 21*(2), 95–103.

Rogers, C. R. (1975). Empathic: An unappreciated way of being. *Counseling Psychologist, 5*(2), 2–10.

Saint Exupéry, A. de. (1971). *The little prince* (K. Woods, Trans.). New York: Harcourt, Brace and World. (Original work published 1943)

Thomas, L. (1983a). *The medusa and the snail: Notes of a biology watcher.* New York: Viking.

Thomas, L. (1983b). *The youngest science: Notes of a medicine-watcher.* New York: Viking.

Titchener, E. B. (1973). *Lectures on the experimental psychology of the thought-processes: Classics in psychology.* New York: Arno Press. (Original work published 1909)

Art: An Occupation With Promise for Developing Empathy

Suzanne M. Peloquin

Key Words: activity analysis • occupational therapy (treatment) • professional–patient relations

Empathy is central to the interactions of occupational therapists who value personal dignity. Persons from various sectors of the behavioral sciences and the medical humanities have proposed that engagement with the arts can develop empathy, an assumption that prompted this inquiry. The observations of artists and art philosophers suggest that the assumption that art may develop empathy is grounded in the kindred natures of the two practices and in the actions that occur when a person engages with a work of art. The assumption that art may develop empathy is grounded in the kinship of the actions common to both practices: response, emotion, and connection. Artists and art philosophers' observations of human practices have uncovered three rules of art that may dispose one toward empathy: reliance on bodily senses, use of metaphor, and occupation by virtual worlds. Analysis of art's potential suggests that a person who would derive empathy from art must (a) use the senses to grasp feeling, (b) stretch the imagination to see a new perspective, and (c) invite an occupation that enhances understanding. Persons who hope to develop empathy must pursue an experience that evokes the fellow feeling that inspires it. Art can offer this experience.

Suzanne M. Peloquin, PhD, OTR, is Professor, Department of Occupational Therapy, School of Allied Health Sciences, The University of Texas Medical Branch at Galveston, 301 University Boulevard, Galveston, Texas 77555-1028, and is Consultant, Department of Occupational Therapy, Transitional Learning Community at Galveston, Galveston, Texas.

This article was accepted for publication August 19, 1995.

Therapists have discussed the importance of empathy in the occupational therapy process (Baum, 1980; King, 1980; Yerxa, 1980), and a select few have engaged in research efforts related to the construct (Christiansen, 1977; Wise & Page, 1980). In an official document that supported this earlier work, the American Occupational Therapy Association (AOTA, 1993a) identified empathy as central to the interactions of occupational therapists. Rogers (1975) described the disposition that is so valued in occupational therapy:

> It means entering the private world of the other and becoming thoroughly at home in it. It involves being sensitive, moment to moment, to the changing felt meanings which flow in the other person, to the fear or rage or tenderness or confusion or whatever, that he or she is experiencing....In some respects it means that you lay aside your self. (p. 3)

Decades ago, May (1939) argued in the behavioral science literature that the artistic experience coaxes persons toward empathy by taking them out of themselves. More currently, the enfranchisement of humanities subjects within a number of medical schools rests on several assumptions, one of them being that art fosters empathy (Charon et al., 1995).

Within the occupational therapy literature, art has been linked with empathy indirectly. The *Essentials and Guidelines for an Accredited Educational Program for the Occupational Therapist* (AOTA, 1993b) recommended a broad foundation of the liberal arts to develop capacities in communication and understanding—constructs linked with empathy. The use of specific works of art has been described as a workable means of sustaining the art of practice and enhancing therapists' understanding of their patients (Peloquin, 1989, 1996).

Art's association with empathy also appears in fiction. Shem's (1981) novel about the depersonalizing force of the medical system showed the effect of art on an intern named Roy Basch. After working for some time at the House of God hospital, Basch recalled:

> I lay on top of my bed and did not sleep. I imagined I felt what the gomers felt: an absence of feeling. I had no idea how bad I might be, but I knew that I could not do what Dr. Sanders had told us to do, to "be with" others. I could not "be with" others, for I was somewhere else, in some cold place. (p. 317)

Friends got Basch away from work for an artistic event, and as one performer mimed the stages of youth, maturity, old age, and death, the intern was touched: "All of a sudden I felt as if a hearing aid for all my senses had been turned on. I was flooded with feeling....A handkerchief was placed in my hand, I blew my nose. I felt a hug" (p. 360). He later thought:

That was a beginning. To repair, to recreate the human took some time....As I began to repair I asked myself what had been missing...I realized that what had been missing was all that I loved. I would be transformed. I'd not leave that country of love again. (p. 363)

This assumption about art's capacity to rekindle sensibility resonates with truth on an intuitive level. May's (1939) hypothesis that art can coax persons toward empathy seems equally plausible. Most assumptions about art, however, lack the clarity and specificity of an articulate argument. Why do the arts invite the assumption that they will awaken a person's sensibilities? What happens during an engagement with art that may yield fellow feeling? Do persons with expertise in the arts express similar views about the potential of art? These questions structured this inquiry.

The Nature of Art and Its Connection With Empathy as Seen in the Literature

The literature on art is vast, reaching back into antiquity and stretching across numerous fields to constitute a wealth of statements. In the face of this abundance, one can scarcely make an assertion about art without knowing that someone has elsewhere or at a different time disclosed another view. Moreover, to speak of art is to minimize the distinctions among the individual arts. Listening to a symphony is an act that differs from reading a novel or contemplating a sketch. Yet the likenesses among these acts—that each is art—make the world of art. When one steps into this world to explore the claim that art develops empathy, one restricts the search minimally.

For this inquiry, the visual and literary arts served as focal points for discussion. The nature of empathy as found in an earlier review of the behavioral science and philosophical literature further narrowed the search to the themes that characterize an empathic encounter: (a) an expression of being there, (b) a turning of the soul, (c) a recognition of both likeness and uniqueness in another, (d) an entry into the other's experience, (e) a connection with the other's feelings, (f) a power to recover from that connection, and (g) a personal enrichment that derives from these actions (Peloquin, 1995).

A sampling of 50 twentieth-century books on art available on a medical school campus that houses a humanities program served as resources. Any text or chapter that promised, by title, to address the aforementioned themes was reviewed. Citations and bibliographies from these first texts enlarged the search to more than 90 books and articles. The citations within this article are a representative sampling of a larger discussion.

A significant association between art and empathy that comes from the literature is that their natures are kindred. Artists and art philosophers identify three actions that works of art elicit from those who produce or appreciate them: (a) response, (b) emotion, and (c) connection. It can be argued that each of these actions resembles the actions of empathy.

Response

Art is known for the response that it prompts. Panofsky (1955) described the receptivity that characterizes this response. A work of art begins with an artist disposed to respond; it culminates in the response of those who appreciate it.

> When a man looks at a tree from the point of view of a carpenter, he will associate it with the various uses to which he might put the wood; and when he looks at it from the point of view of an ornithologist he will associate it with the birds that might nest in it....Only he who simply and wholly abandons himself to the object of his perception will experience it aesthetically. (p. 11)

Art invites an immersion in some reality for the sake of understanding it.

An artist is also responsive to the artistic medium. Suppose that the cycles of natural events catch an artist's attention. Depending on the medium used, the artist will respond differently:

> A pencil creates objects by circumscribing their shape with a line. A brush, which creates broader spots, may suggest a disk-shaped patch of color. In the medium of clay or stone the best equivalent of roundness is a sphere. A dancer will create it by running a circular path, spinning around his own axis, or by arranging a group of dancers in a circle. (Arnheim, 1966a, p. 92)

In the making of art, the response that occurs is an interaction among artist, art–object, and medium. In the appreciation of art, the response is an interaction among audience, artist, and art–object. Both responses are interplays between thoughts and feelings. Carpenter (1919) thus said that artistic endeavors extend a basic human activity: "Within ourselves there is a continual movement outwards from Feeling towards Thought, and then to Action" (p. 15).

The movement is not linear, as Edman (1939) explained: "Anyone, indeed, who has ever written poetry knows how a poem often begins in the mind as a kind of cadence with a hardly specified meaning" (p. 68). Gilmour (1986) shared Edman's sense of how meaning develops:

> It is a misconception of the creative act to think of it as arising from a clear-cut intention of the artist, as if the materials employed were a mere means of expression....A more realistic picture of the creative process is that after a certain amount of work has been done, the artist looks at the result, considers how to go on, and then modifies the piece as seems appropriate. (p. 16)

When an artist begins to create, so does a responsive search for meaning. When that search culminates in a work of art, a new search—for the meaning of color, cadence, or image—begins with the audience.

A work of art is so responsive in its becoming that it seems to be alive. Dillard (1982) saw life in the medium:

> One does not choose a prose, or a handling of paint, as a fitting tool for a given task, the way one chooses a 5/16 wrench to loosen a 5/16 bolt. Rather—and rather creepily—the prose "secretes" the book. (p. 124)

But Booth (1988) argued that the medium merely prompts creative action. It is the artist's engagement, he said, that turns art into something human: "To dwell with a creative task for as long as is required to perform it well means that one tends to become the work—at least to some degree" (p. 51). To dwell with a work for as long as it takes to appreciate it demands a similar engagement. Art evokes a response that is deep and personal.

Empathy is known for a response similar to that found in art. One who empathizes enters into an exchange that shapes understanding of another's reality. Empathy calls for a receptivity to and active grasp of the situation and feelings of someone else. An empathic encounter is an interplay among a person who empathizes, a person who seeks understanding, and an event that prompts their connection. Like in art, the exchange of empathy moves back and forth from feeling to thought to action. When one person empathizes with another, the action is deep and personally responsive. The parallels between art and empathy are striking.

Emotion

The response that art evokes is often emotional. Emotion is thus the second characteristic in art that suggests its kinship with empathy. Langer (1953) called art the "envisagement of feeling" (p. 380) because many persons seem to turn to it for its emotionality. Edman (1939) described the intensity of the open-faced expression rendered in art:

> The artist, be he poet, painter, sculptor, or architect, does something to objects, the poet and novelist do something to events, that compel the eye to stop and find pleasure in the beholding, the ear to hear for the sheer sake of listening, the mind to attend. (p. 17)

Such intensity of expression evokes strong feelings:

> Suppose someone has studied certain facts, say, the physics of gravitation. He may have thoroughly understood the theoretical and practical consequences of the phenomenon. One day, suddenly, he is seized by the experience of what gravitation actually does to life and nature. He acknowledges the sensation of being pulled downward and he feels the same pull in all the animate and inanimate

things about him....Such sensitivity is closely related to, or perhaps identical with, art. (Arnheim, 1966b, p. 342)

Because works of art customarily rouse feelings, Edman (1939) called them truancies from rational practices. He argued that literature teaches fellow feeling more clearly than life does. Dillard (1982) agreed:

> In daily life we never understand each other, neither complete clairvoyance nor complete confessional exists. We know each other approximately, by external signs....But people in a novel can be understood completely by the reader, if the novelist wishes; their inner as well as their outer life can be exposed. (p. 47)

Goodman (1976a) said that although it would be absurd to see art as an emotional orgy, persons are so open to feelings in art that they often welcome works that arouse negative emotions of fear or disgust, accepting these as natural expressions of humanity.

At the end of the nineteenth century, Tolstoy (1960) argued art's responsibility in terms of feeling. He said, "The task for art to accomplish is to make that feeling of brotherhood and love of one's neighbor, now attained only by the best members of society, the customary feeling and the instinct of all men" (p. 190). Art's validation of emotions is one way of fostering fellowship.

Like art, empathy affirms emotionality. Empathy demands a sensitivity that stops, attends, and then grasps the feelings of someone else. The heightened sense of another's emotion may be seen as the turning that is called *soulful* in the literature on empathy (Buber, 1965). A fundamental aim of the empathic encounter, like the fundamental responsibility of art, is to make the feeling of brotherhood more customary.

Connection

The third characteristic action that art and empathy share is connection. Art both asks and helps persons to make connections with others. For this reason, Gilmour (1986) called visual works rehearsals for taking new perspectives: "Once we have experienced a Cézanne landscape, for example, we begin to see our own surroundings with his eyes....After intense involvement with art works we return to the world with new eyes" (p. 22).

Artists introduce their audiences to others whose views may differ:

> One moves with [artists] in lands where one has never been, experiences loves one has never known. And this entrance into lives wider and more various than our own in turn enables us more nicely to appreciate and more intensely to live the lives we do not know. (Edman, 1939, p. 84)

Because of its capacity to bring strangers together, Dewey

(1934) saw art's moral purpose: "To remove prejudice, do away with the scales that keep the eye from seeing, tear away the veils due to wont and custom, perfect the power to perceive" (p. 365).

In spite of its emotionality and its intensity, art facilitates connections by allowing a safe distance. Wind (1985) explained:

> Art is an exercise of the imagination, engaging and detaching us at the same time: it makes us participate in what it presents, and yet presents it as an aesthetic fiction. From that twofold root—participation and fiction—art draws its power to enlarge our vision by carrying us beyond the actual, and to deepen our experience by compassion. (p. 24)

Bruner (1966) believed that even one such venture stirs an appetite for more. "Having sensed connectedness," he said, "one is impelled to seek more of it" (p. 73).

Empathy, too, makes connections. Empathy requires a participation in the life of another that is personal and without prejudice. It is a kind of participation that is both engagement and detachment because overengagement would crush the capacity to help. Empathic connections, like those made in art, deepen one person's sense of another's reality through appreciation and compassion.

The evidence of a kinship between art and empathy rests on three actions common to both practices: response, emotion, and connection. This likeness of action suggests that those who would enhance their capacity to empathize in health care practice might learn from art how to respond, feel, and make meaningful connections.

The Specific Rules of Art That Promise to Develop Empathy

As they discuss that which causes response, emotion, and connection to occur, artists and art philosophers make observations that further clarify the hypothesis that art can develop empathy. These observations begin within a discussion of human practices.

Whether in the realm of art, science, or health care, MacIntyre (1984) defined practice as any coherent form of socially established activity within which goods internal to that activity are realized in the course of meeting its standards. An example may clarify his meaning. Chess players can increase their capacity to solve problems—an internal good—as they master the rules and steps of the game. MacIntyre elaborated:

> We call them internal goods for two reasons: first...because we can only specify them in terms of chess or some other game of that specific kind and by means of examples from such games; and secondly because they can only be identified and recognized by the experience of participating in the practice in question. (pp. 188–189)

MacIntyre's (1984) conceptualization of internal

goods is apt for this discussion because empathy seems to be an internal good that may follow engagement with art. Those who discuss art cite certain aspects with such regularity that they emerge as rules. Three of these rules may dispose a person toward empathy: reliance on bodily senses, use of metaphor, and occupation by virtual worlds. Each rule warrants further discussion in terms of its potential.

Reliance on Bodily Senses

Art relies on the senses. Arnheim (1969) proposed that a person who paints, writes, composes, or dances, thinks with the senses. He also described the confluence of cognition and sensation that occurs in most persons:

> As I open my eyes, I find myself surrounded by a given world: the sky with its clouds, the moving waters of the lake, the wind-swept dunes, the window, my study, my desk, my body....Through that world roams the glance, directed by attention, focusing the narrow range of sharpest vision now on this, now on that spot, following the flight of a distant sea gull, scanning a tree to explore its shape. This eminently active performance is what is meant by visual perception. (p. 14)

Because of its intelligent aspect, Arnheim renamed perception *visual thinking*. Artists engage their visual thinking capacities and ask their audiences to do the same.

As one example, artists read muscular behaviors at their emotional levels and re-create them to show the expressive nature of persons. Everyday total body movements become expressions in art: "Muscular behavior such as grasping, yielding, lifting, straightening, smoothing, loosening, bending, running, stopping, seem to produce mental resonance effects constantly" (Arnheim, 1966b, p. 69). Arnheim (1966b) thus asked persons to note the joyful abandon in the high-stepping bodies of Matisse's dancers and to see oppressive fatigue in Picasso's rendering of a woman at her ironing. In addition to the dancing and ironing that they portray, these bodies express emotion. One who engages in visual thinking about these bodily movements can derive a deeper understanding of what a high-stepping kick or a bending back can mean.

This rule of relying on the senses is not restricted to the visual arts. Wilde (1970) claimed that "it is Literature that shows us the body in its swiftness and the soul in its unrest" (p. 130). The expressive gestures in Tolstoy's (1981) work are fine examples, particularly at that point when the title character lies near death:

> "But what is the real thing?" he asked himself and grew quiet, listening. Just then he felt someone kissing his hand. He opened his eyes and looked at his son. He grieved for him. His wife came in and

went up to him. She gazed at him with an open mouth, with un-
wiped tears on her nose and cheeks, with a look of despair on her
face. He grieved for her. (p. 132)

No matter where in art one finds bodily expressions, one
hones sensitivity in grasping their meaning (Panofsky,
1995).

Art builds on a common understanding that derives
from the bodily senses. Paradoxically, however, art affirms the idiosyncratic character of human expression.
Most artists, like Goodman (1976a), readily acknowledge their work as one way of seeing: "The eye comes
always ancient to its work, obsessed by its own past and
by insinuations of ear, nose, tongue, finger, heart, and
brain" (p. 7). Because art is so open to various interpretations, it proves human subjectivity.

Art's rule of relying on the senses may foster empathy by reminding therapists to scrutinize bodily expressions for their universal meaning. Therapists who master
this rule might see others more fully, attending to the
meaning of their gestures and intimations. A reaching
hand or whining voice might be read as communications
of familiar sentiments. Treatments might then include a
hopeful nod or caring touch in a nonverbal reciprocity of
feeling.

Art's rule of relying on the senses may also foster
empathy by reminding therapists of the singularity of personal views. After repeated encounters with subjective
portrayals, therapists might see the tenuousness of book-
learned theories. Claims to professional objectivity or better knowledge might yield to collaborations that include
the patient's perspective. Therapists sensitized through art
might act on art's lesson that any human reality implies a
point of view.

Use of Metaphor

A second rule that promises to develop empathy is art's
use of metaphor to convey meaning. When using metaphor, an artist consciously likens two entities. Goodman
(1976a) discussed metaphors in the context of travel. A
metaphor, he said, has a home realm in which it dwells as
a fact; an artist coaxes words or symbols into alien realms
where they become "calculated category-mistakes" (p. 79).
The word *pistol*, for example, dwells in the realm of fire-
arms as a fact. It becomes a calculated category-mistake
when placed in the alien realm of the comment, "She's a
real pistol!"

Gilmour (1986) saw the visual metaphor of New
York City in Mondrian's painting *Broadway Boogie Woogie*,
with its grid-like bands and vivid shapes filling the canvas.
Metaphor demands imagination. After engaging with

Mondrian's metaphor, a person might more readily see
the rhythmic design in most cities.

Because metaphors make fresh connections, Gilmour
(1986) argued that this mental activity stretches the capacity to understand. Booth (1988) argued more boldly
that metaphor is an invitation to intimacy. He said that
when Shakespeare had King Lear cry out, "Take physic,
pomp" (p. 190), he pulled others into his perspective:

No matter how strongly I might object to having my mind turned
to compare the flow of wealth to flowing feces, the command issued
by the metaphor will have been obeyed even as I understand it. A
part of my mind has thus been shaped into an intense active discussion about the gross parallels between taking a physic and curing
pomp's indifference to poverty and suffering. (p. 190)

Some persons may not agree that they should purge their
lives of proud displays. But they must know Shakespeare's
meaning before they disagree. Understanding starts with
this grasp of meaning.

Mastery of metaphor might dispose a person to empathize. A therapist grown accustomed to meanings
found in metaphor might learn how disability affects a
patient by asking, "What is this like for you?" Upon hearing that a patient feels like so many pounds of meat, a
therapist might imagine the pain in such reduction. Therapists at ease with the travel of metaphor might more
readily visit the alien realms of their patients.

Repeatedly exposed to metaphors that stretch their
imagination, therapists might see humdrum in mindless
routines and lock-step protocols. They might liken therapy to gardening or friendship and thus personalize their
practice. Having found the worth of calculated category-
mistakes, they might seek dissonant views as a source of
fresh connections.

Occupation by Virtual Worlds

The third rule of art that may develop empathy is its call
to inhabit virtual worlds. Goodman (1976b) affirmed
the reality of fictional worlds: "Worldmaking as we know
it always starts from the world that is already on hand;
the making is a remaking" (p. 6). Fictional works seem
real, and most readers engage with art because they find
it meaningful.

In fact, works of art offer a coherence not so obvious
in reality. Edman (1939) thus proposed that "the place to
seek for reality is not in some metaphysical formula, but
in the unimpeachable realities in works of art" (p. 57).
Booth (1988) cast the process of engaging with art in
terms of occupation:

When a story "works," when we like it well enough to listen to it
again and tell it over and over to ourselves and friends...it occupies

us in a curiously intense way. The pun in "occupy" is useful here. We are occupied in the sense of filling our time with the story—its time takes over our time. And we are occupied in the sense of being taken over, colonized: occupied by a foreign imaginary world. (p. 139)

Such occupation allows this discovery: "We find in art objects qualities in which the great world and its parts seem often wanting: human significance, human order, reason, mind, causality, boundary, harmony, perfection, coherence, purity, purpose, and permanence" (Dillard, 1982, p. 176).

Repeated sojourns into virtual worlds can develop empathy. Through art, therapists can learn about life from a number of scenes and characters. They can step into experiences with illness, disability, and occupation, using the realities of fiction as opportunities for observation, reflection, and understanding. They can learn from fictional caregivers how they succeed or fail. And in doing all of this, therapists can rehearse the call of empathy—to walk in another's shoes.

The comments of artists and art philosophers give clarity and support to the otherwise vague assumption that art might foster empathy. It can be hypothesized that reliance on bodily senses, use of metaphor, and occupation by virtual worlds can prepare therapists for the sensing, imagining, and understanding that structure empathy.

Discussion

This inquiry may be seen as an analysis of those aspects of art that promise to develop empathy. Whether they practice as clinicians, educators, or administrators, therapists who hope to foster empathy may find in this search a reason for using the arts.

Two disclaimers need to be made, however. No one can guarantee that *exposure* to works of art will foster empathy. The strongest suggestion from the literature is that regular engagement in the actions of art may rehearse the actions of empathy. To derive the internal good of empathy, a person must practice the rules of art. The requisite practice thus consists of (a) using the senses to grasp feeling, (b) stretching the imagination to see a new perspective, and (c) inviting an occupation that allows understanding. Only after such an involvement might a person enhance the capacity to respond, feel, or make connections.

A second disclaimer associates with the work of art. In a culture enchanted by rationality, artists can lose their evocative power. Arnheim (1969) saw the dilemma: "Nor are pedantry, sterility, and mechanization found only in the sciences; they are equally present in the arts" (p. 296).

Wind (1985) presented a jarring image of artists as technicians:

Often they seem to act in their studios as if they were in the laboratory, performing a series of controlled experiments in the hope of arriving at a valid scientific solution. And when these astringent exercises are exhibited, they reduce the spectator to an observer who watches the artist's latest excursion with interest, but without vital participation. (p. 21)

If a work is a technical exercise that fails to evoke a participation, it is not likely that response, emotion, or connection will occur.

Summary

Empathy is valued in occupational therapy as an attitude that affirms human dignity. A number of persons from within the behavioral sciences have suggested that the artistic experience can develop empathy. The vagueness of their suggestions prompted this inquiry and literature review guided by three questions: (a) Why do the arts invite the assumption that they will awaken a person's sensibilities? (b) What happens during an engagement with art that may yield fellow feeling? and (c) Do persons with expertise in the arts express similar views about the potential of art?

The answers to these questions clarify the assumption that art may develop empathy. Artists and philosophers suggest that art rouses a person's sensibilities because it invites response, emotion, and connection. The derivative suggestion is that art can be a rehearsal for empathy because empathy's actions are similar to those of art. The literature clarifies this second assumption by describing three rules of art: the reliance on bodily senses, the use of metaphor, and the occupation by virtual worlds. These rules may dispose therapists to empathize in practice.

This analysis of art's potential began with an observation from Shem's (1981) novel about the House of God hospital. At the story's end, Basch expressed his sadness over the lingering bitterness that followed his year of internship in a depersonalized environment. When his fiancée suggested that he might be a better person because of his experience among the hopelessly demented and dying, Basch asked how. She replied:

This might have been the only thing that could have awakened you. Your whole life has been a growing from the outside, mastering the challenges that others have set for you. Now, finally, you might just be growing from inside yourself. It can be a whole new world, Roy, I know it. A whole new life. (p. 418)

Her comment goes to the heart of this inquiry because there is no escaping this fact: Empathy requires a growing from inside the self. A person who hopes to be empathic must pursue an experience that awakens the sense of fellowship. Artists and art philosophers suggest that such an awakening can occur through art. ▲

Acknowledgment

The research for this article originated within a portion of a dissertation entitled Art in Practice: When Art Becomes Caring, completed in partial fulfillment of requirements for a doctoral degree granted in 1991 by the Institute for the Medical Humanities of the University of Texas Medical Branch, Galveston, Texas.

References

American Occupational Therapy Association. (1993a). Core values and attitudes of occupational therapy practice. *American Journal of Occupational Therapy, 47,* 1085–1086.

American Occupational Therapy Association. (1993b). *Essentials and guidelines for an accredited educational program for the occupational therapist.* Rockville, MD: American Occupational Therapy Association.

Arnheim, R. (1966a). Growth. In E. W. Eisner & D. W. Ecker (Eds.), *Readings and art education* (pp. 85–96). Waltham, MA: Blaisdell.

Arnheim, R. (1966b). *Toward a psychology of art.* Berkeley, CA: University of California Press.

Arnheim, R. (1969). *Visual thinking.* Berkeley, CA: University of California Press.

Baum, C. M. (1980). Eleanor Clarke Slagle lecture—Occupational therapists put care in the health system. *American Journal of Occupational Therapy, 34,* 505–516.

Booth, W. C. (1988). *The company we keep: An ethics of fiction.* Berkeley: University of California Press.

Bruner, J. (1966). *On knowing: Essays for the left hand.* Cambridge, MA: Belknap Press.

Buber, M. (1965). *Between man and man.* New York: Macmillan.

Carpenter, E. (1919). *The act of creation: Essays on the self and its powers.* London: George Allen & Unwin.

Charon, R., Banks, J. T., Connelly, J. E., Hawkins, A. H., Hunter, K. N., Jones, A. H., Montello, M., & Poirier, S. (1995). Literature and medicine: Contributions to clinical practice. *American College of Physicians, 122,* 599–619.

Christiansen, C. H. (1977). Measuring empathy in occupational therapy students. *American Journal of Occupational Therapy, 31,* 19–22.

Dewey, J. (1934). *Art as experience.* New York: Pedigree.

Dillard, A. (1982). *Living by fiction.* New York: Harper & Row.

Edman, I. (1939). *Arts and the man: A short introduction to aesthetics.* New York: Norton.

Gilmour, J. (1986). *Picturing the world.* Albany, NY: State University of New York Press.

Goodman, N. (1976a). *Language of art: An approach to a theory of symbols.* Indianapolis: Hackett.

Goodman, N. (1976b). *Ways of worldmaking.* Indianapolis: Hackett.

King, L. J. (1980). Creative caring. *American Journal of Occupational Therapy, 34,* 522–528.

Langer, S. (1953). *Feeling and form: A theory of art.* New York: Scribner.

MacIntyre, A. (1984). *After virtue: A study in moral theory.* Terre-Haute, IN: University of Notre Dame Press.

May, R. (1939). *The art of counseling.* New York: Abingdon.

Panofsky, E. (1955). *Meaning in the visual arts.* Garden City, NJ: Doubleday/Anchor.

Peloquin, S. M. (1989). Sustaining the art of practice in occupational therapy. *American Journal of Occupational Therapy, 43,* 219–226.

Peloquin, S. M. (1995). The fullness of empathy: Reflections and illustrations. *American Journal of Occupational Therapy, 49,* 24–31.

Peloquin, S. M. (1996). Using the arts to enhance confluent learning. *American Journal of Occupational Therapy, 50,* 148–151.

Rogers, C. R. (1975). Empathic: An unappreciated way of being. *Counseling Psychologist, 5,* 2–10.

Shem, S. (1981). *The house of God.* New York: Dell.

Tolstoy, L. (1960). *What is art?* (A. Maude, Trans.). New York: Liberal Arts Press.

Tolstoy, L. (1981). *The death of Ivan Ilyich.* (L. Solotaroff, Trans.). New York: Bantam.

Wilde, O. (1970). *The soul of man under socialism.* New York: Harper & Row.

Wind, E. (1985). *Art and anarchy.* Evanston, IL: Northwestern University Press.

Wise, B. L., & Page, M. S. (1980). Empathy levels of occupational therapy students. *American Journal of Occupational Therapy, 34,* 676–679.

Yerxa, E. J. (1980). Occupational therapy's role in creating a future climate of caring. *American Journal of Occupational Therapy, 34,* 529–534.

The Patient–Therapist Relationship: Beliefs That Shape Care

Suzanne M. Peloquin

Key Words: competence, professional • social environment

The results of a previous inquiry suggest that three images of occupational therapists dominate patients' stories about them: the images of technician, parent, and collaborator or friend. These ways of being in practice can be said to reflect the various understandings that therapists have about how to enact the profession's commitment to both competence and caring. When therapists act as technicians or authoritarian parents, patients register their disappointment over a valuation of competence that excludes caring actions.

In a more current inquiry into the climate of caring, patients and caregivers reflect about the current health care system and identify three societal constructs that shape a preference for competence over caring: (a) emphasis on the rational fixing of the health care problem, (b) overreliance on methods and protocols, and (c) a health care system driven by business, efficiency, and profit. Occupational therapists who are concerned about complaints that the health care system is increasingly uncaring might benefit from a consideration of the extent to which societal beliefs shape the manner in which they care.

O ccupational therapists can be with patients in many ways that reflect their various understandings of what it means to be competent and caring. Because the beliefs of a profession shape a therapist's sense of what it means to give care, the beliefs about competence and caring found in the occupational therapy tradition have warranted consideration (Peloquin, 1990). Three images of how occupational therapists act in practice dominate patients' stories: the images of technician, parent, and collaborator or friend. When therapists act as technicians or authoritarian parents, patients cast them negatively in stories that reflect their disappointment. When acting in either of these manners, therapists seem to value the competence articulated within the professional literature more than they value the caring aspects of *relationship* (Peloquin, 1990). Both of these enactments, however, reflect some understanding of what it means to care. The technical therapist, equating expertise with care, values the best method and the successful outcome. The parental therapist manipulates the decisions and methods that are in the patient's best interests and sees this action as caring. In each of these images of care, the therapist's competence dominates the encounter.

If choosing how to be among patients is a matter of some consideration, it follows that a number of societal beliefs and expectations also shape a therapist's choice. Those beliefs are the subject of this discussion. It seems apt for occupational therapists to consider the societal forces that surround practice. As Yerxa (1980) said, "Occupational therapy, which began in a climate of caring, has been influenced in its practice by social change" (p. 532). It is a growing truism that the current health care system is now perceived as "not oriented to the human being" (Baum, 1980, p. 514). What causes this disorientation to persons? King (1980) suggested that any sense of the meaning of caring is an intermingling of personal, professional, *and* societal beliefs. Any lack of caring that derives from a preferential valuation of competence must also reflect such an intermingling.

Nature and Scope of the Inquiry

This article constitutes part of a larger inquiry into the challenge of creating a climate of caring. Conducted between January 1990 and September 1991, the inquiry considered the following: (a) personal narratives that describe impersonal treatment; (b) the historical events and societal constructs that have shaped the patient–helper relationship; (c) empathy and the manner in which helpers learn to be empathic; (d) the nature, practice, and experience of art; and (f) the proposition that empathy might be cultivated through the use of art. Each step of the inquiry required an extensive literature review from which important themes emerged. These themes were

Suzanne M. Peloquin, PhD, OTR, is Associate Professor of Occupational Therapy, School of Allied Health Sciences, J-28, 11th and Mechanic Street, University of Texas Medical Branch at Galveston, Galveston, Texas 77555–1028.

This article was accepted for publication June 4, 1993.

then subjected to the reflection, analysis, and synthesis characteristic of studies in the medical humanities.

A number of phenomenological narratives about the impersonal treatment of patients served as subjects for an earlier discussion (Peloquin, 1993). That discussion produced a descriptive profile of those behaviors to which patients refer when they use the term *depersonalizing*. The central complaint found within those narratives was that when practitioners act impersonally their behaviors are discouraging. Patients say that helpers fail to see illness and disability as emotional events charged with personal meaning. They fail to attend to the experiences of patients; instead, they establish a distance that diminishes them. They withhold information, they use brusque manners, and they misuse their powers. They are insensitive, silent, and aloof. Patients conclude that their helpers may treat them, but they do not treat them well.

Alongside these descriptive narratives were a number not included in the discussion on depersonalization because they were more reflective than descriptive: (a) those written by patients who consider the beliefs that may cause their helpers to behave carelessly; (b) those written by caregivers who, after their own bout with illness and impersonal treatment, discuss societal expectations; and (c) those written by helpers who ponder the difficulties of caring. These reflections offer cues about the societal constructs that may have a hand in shaping care, and, as cues, they constitute assumptions that can direct further research.

This discussion does not address concerns in practice such as those that Bailey (1990) described as the "harmful variables" that cause therapists to leave the field (p. 23). Staff shortages, large caseloads, red tape, excessive paperwork, lack of job status, chronic conditions of the patient population, lack of respect for occupational therapy by other professionals, stress and overload, and the need to justify treatment also shape decisions about the manner in which helpers will choose to care. Many of these negative variables, although not the specific focus of this inquiry, can also be said to associate with the societal beliefs that are the subject of this discussion.

The Connections That Mean Care

A number of stories do portray helpers as caring persons who offer patients equal measures of competence and caring (Peloquin, 1989; Peloquin, 1990). These stories suggest that caring attitudes, gestures, and words give patients the courage to face illness and disability.

Pekkanen (1988) treated a 14-year-old boy whose electrical accident had warranted amputation of his legs; Pekkanen willed himself to feel the boy's injury from the inside out. He then understood:

> He was a tall, rangy black kid from the inner city and had been a very good junior high school basketball player. All he ever wanted to be was a basketball player, and I think that the young man took

this news with more hurt, more disappointment, and more disbelief than any child I can remember. . . . I think it was one of the most crushing truths to come to a young man that I have ever seen. (p. 126)

A caring attitude can encourage patients. Lee (1987), a patient hospitalized with cancer, felt care in this small gesture:

> As I slept a nurse took the cloth wrapping off a sterile instrument. He smoothed out the material. He painted with a blue flow pen a moon face with wide eyes and an enormous crescent smile. He climbed over my bed. He climbed over my plants and hung this banner down from my window, using the extra-wide masking tape. It was the first thing I saw in the morning. (p. 111)

Patients also draw courage from caring words. Benziger (1969) remembered the encouragement that she took from this conversation with an occupational therapist:

> "You know, you go at your work too hard, too fast, too desperately—and too frenetically."
> "I guess I do, but that's the way I feel. Time stands still for me now, it is endless, and yet if I have something to do, I get the sense that there will not be time enough to finish it, or that someone will stop me."
> She said, "You are an intelligent person, and you will help yourself to get well quickly." "You know," I answered, "you're the first person who has mentioned intelligence versus non-intelligence, instead of sanity. You make me feel like a human being." I was grateful. I should not forget her. (p. 49)

The directness and the proffered confidence held in these words meant concern to Benziger; she would call this therapist *friend*.

Sarason's (1985) point of view is no doubt the most helpful. At the very least, he said, practitioners can *try*. Patients, he says, mostly ask helpers to try "in ways that say 'I am trying to understand because I want to be helpful.' It is those manifestations that are experienced as caring and compassionate, even though they may be more or less ineffective" (p. 188). And when "a patient, whether terminal or not, draws courage—courage to live or courage to die—from the man who stands at his bedside" (Hodgins, 1964, p. 843), surely they both feel the magic of care.

If practitioners can be both competent and caring among their patients, what societal beliefs cause them to act otherwise? Three constructs surface within the reflections of patients and practitioners as shaping forces that compromise caring expressions: (a) an emphasis on the rational fixing of problems; (b) an overreliance on methods and protocols; and (c) a health care provision system that is driven by business, efficiency, and profit.

The Emphasis on Rational Fixing

One societal belief that compromises caring actions is the emphasis on solving discrete health care problems in a logical and rational manner. When Hodgins wrote in 1964 after his stroke, he found a particular form of disregard at the heart of the problem. He described this picture of how the patient and the caregiver perceive illness:

936

> In stroke two basic sets of assumptions could govern treatment. One set proceeds from what the patient perceives or thinks he perceives; the other comes from what the doctor knows or thinks he knows. The two are very different sets of things. (p. 842)

Many health care narratives hold similar pictures, with helpers governing some aspects of care while neglecting others that their patients value. Sir Dominic Corrigan, a physician, argued as long as a century ago that the trouble with doctors is "not that they don't know enough, but that they don't see enough" (cited in Taylor, 1972, p. 6).

Van Eys (1988), also a physician, has regretted the hemisected worldview in which "diseases become problems, and patients become dissected into such problems" (p. 21). Patients resent this narrowness of focus because it feels uncaring. They complain that practitioners address their disease, the physiology and the mechanism of their bodies and dysfunctions, but not the experience of illness and unease, not its meaning, and surely not their feelings.

Disregard for parts of persons disturbs Murphy (1987), an anthropologist who wrote of his own disabling illness: "The full subjective states of the patient are of little concern in the medical model of disability, which holds that the problem arises wholly from some atomic or physiological disorder and is correctible by standard modes of therapy—drugs, surgery, radiation, or whatever" (p. 88). Sacks (1983), a neurologist who experienced impersonal care, considered this splitting insane:

> the madness of the last three centuries, the madness which so many of us—as individuals—go through, and by which all of us are tempted. It is the Newtonian-Lockean-Cartesian view—variously paraphrased in medicine, biology, politics, industry, etc.—which reduces men to machines, automata, puppets, dolls, blank tablets, formulae, ciphers, systems, and reflexes. (p. 205)

Sarton (1988) remembered in her journal that after a stroke she was made to feel like "so many pounds of meat, filled with potentially interesting mechanical parts and neurochemical combinations" (p. 106).

Leder (1984) argued while in medical school that a person is never so many pounds of meat, that the human body is "not a mere extrinsic machine but our living center" (p. 34). Paradoxically, however, it seems that the body, so prized in this narrow view of illness, matters little on a day-to-day basis. Most persons, said Leder, ignore the body until it malfunctions. Then when they are ill, they beg some practitioner to fix the complex mechanism that has disrupted the flow of their personal lives. And the picture of health care practice that one then sees is "an ironic fulfillment of Cartesian dualism—a mind (namely, that of the doctor) runs a passive and extrinsic body (that of the patient)" (p. 35). The image offered by Jourard (1964), a psychologist, illuminates this Orwellian disjunction:

> Each patient lies in his own cubicle, and there are attached to him all kinds of wires, connected to his brain, his muscles, his viscera. Every time these wires, which are actually electronic pick-ups, transmit signals to a computer indicating that the bladder is too

full, a bowel stuffed, and patient hungry or in pain, before you could blink an eye, the computer sends signals to different kinds of apparatus which empty the bowel and bladder, fill the stomach, scratch the itch, massage the back and so on. We could even mount the bed on a slowly moving belt; the patient gets in at one end, and four or six days later his bed reaches the exit and the patient is healed—we hope. (p. 138)

If this reduction is a prevalent view, is it fair to expect practitioners to think divergently, to routinely see and treat a self embodied instead of a body? If the general population views the body as a mechanism controlled by higher functions, as something that one has instead of who one is, why the surprise that practitioners engage only their rational functions in practice? If imagining patient experiences, sensing patient needs, and expressing personal feelings seem actions incongruent with fixing, practitioners are quite reasonable in underusing these so-called lower functions. What is the problem, then, with treating bodies when they need fixing?

Most narratives answer that "when a patient appears as a physiological mechanism, the doctor may neglect personal communication in favor of the immediate scientific task at hand" (Leder, 1984, p. 36). The preference for fixing makes it easier for a helper to neglect feelings, easier to justify being silent, curt, or aloof. The resulting problem is impersonal care. Any caregiver can focus narrowly on fixing. Gebolys (1990) remembered this incident:

> A male therapist came in whistling and cheerfully setting up his equipment. He stuck the breathing tube into my mouth and told me to "breathe" which I did while he walked around the room admiring my flowers, gazing out the window and remarking what a lovely day it was. (p. 13)

Mattingly (1991) gave occupational therapists pause for reflection when she argued that "therapists can come to reduce their practice to a manipulation of the physical body, forgetting how much their interventions are directed to a person's life" (p. 986). Parham (1987) argued that there are such situations in occupational therapy when

> time, energy, and money are funneled into treating one small part of the total problem, a part that may be insignificant in comparison with complexities that are more difficult to understand but that have a profound impact on the life situation of the patient being served. (p. 556)

Schultz and Schkade (1992) shared a similar concern: "The current demand for therapists to base occupational therapy on acquisition of functional skills . . . may actually limit the contribution of occupational therapy and may deny patients the opportunity to make vital changes in their occupational adaptation process" (p. 918). Certainly a patient's poem, "Some Other Day" (McClay, 1977), presents an occupational therapist bent on partial fixing:

> Preserve me from the occupational therapist, God
> She means well, but I'm too busy to make baskets. . . .
> "Please, open your eyes," the therapist says;
> You don't want to sleep the day away."
> She wants to know what I used to do,

Knit? Crochet?
Yes, I did those things, and cooked and cleaned, and raised
five children and had things happen to me.
Beautiful things, terrible things,
I need to think about them, rearrange them on the shelves of
my mind.
The therapist is showing me glittery beads.
She asks if I might like to make jewelry.
She's a dear child and she means well,
So I tell her I might.
Some other day. (pp. 107–108)

The consequence of a strong commitment to rational fixing—of the disease, the body, or the dysfunction—is a disregard that feels careless. And although practitioners mean well, physician–educator Anthony Moore (1978) acknowledged the problem: "Professions tend to be right in what they affirm and wrong in what they ignore" (p. 3).

The Reliance on Method and Protocol

A second societal belief that compromises caring is an overreliance on the instruments of health care practice: the techniques, procedures, and modalities that solve the problem. When they are ill, patients seek concern in addition to solutions. They grieve that in health care practice they find something else. Hodgins (1964) regretted the find:

For the physician, of course, it must have been wonderful, indeed, when true specifics began to arrive on the scene to supplant beef, iron, and wine or syrup of hypophosphates. . . . As so-called science more and more enters medicine, the heedless or routine physician will be accordingly tempted to withdraw his humanity and wait for specifics. (p. 843)

Hodgins considered the specifics needed for cure and the humanity needed for care different but inseparable aspects of care. Flagg (1923), a physician who practiced at the turn of the century, agreed; he regretted "the unwise employment of laboratory methods to the exclusion of personal attention" (p. 5).

When a drug or a procedure suffices, a practitioner may think less about the need to make meaningful connections with the patient. The problem becomes clear in Barbara Peabody's (1986) recollection of an incident that occurred during her son's hospitalization for acquired immunodeficiency syndrome (AIDS):

Peter woke at two A.M., just as the intern was about to give him an injection in his left thigh.
"What do you have there?" Peter asked.
"What do you care?" the intern snapped back.
"I care very much, and I hope that's not pentamidine."
"What if it is?" the intern asked insolently.
"Because if it is, I'm not supposed to get it anymore," Peter replied. "I think you better check my chart and you'll see that it was discontinued on Monday."
"Oh, no, the orders are still on your chart."
"I'm sure they're not," Peter insisted. "Go back and read them again, you'll see that I'm right."
The intern left the room and never returned. (p. 51)

Reiser (1980) told the following story about helpers whose reliance on protocol precluded personal attention. A woman hospitalized with a diagnosis of acute granulo-

cytic leukemia and severe anemia agreed to an aggressive course of chemotherapy that made her quite ill. She was discharged after remission, and when she was readmitted 4 months later she refused chemotherapy. The staff decided that if she continued to refuse this treatment, she would be discharged Against Medical Advice. She refused and was discharged. Reiser's perception was that she had "stepped out of the established 'system' and had to be punished for it" (p. 146).

Sacks (1983) rejected the argument that helpers must use *only* treatments or protocols. When facing surgery, he wondered,

What sort of man would Swan be? I knew he was a good surgeon, but it was not the surgeon but the person that I would stand in relation to, or, rather, the man in whom, I hoped, the surgeon and the person would be wholly fused. (p. 92)

Cassell (1985), another physician, shared a similar belief: "Doctors who lack developed personal powers are inadequately trained. . . . Doctors are themselves instruments of patient care" (p. 1).

When they are effective, however, methods and protocols take the upper hand. Helpers side with what works, so that a challenge to the procedure also threatens them. Martha Lear (1980) remembered the upshot of such an identification when her husband Hal, a urologist, requested a milder painkiller: "The resident got angry. He said, 'There is a medication ordered for pain for you. If you want it, you can have it. If not, you'll get nothing.' And he walked out" (p. 41). But patients, wrote the physician Pellegrino (1979), do not want practitioners to fuse with their skills: "Physicians have a medical education, an M.D. degree, a set of skills, knowledge, prestige, titles. They possess many things by which they mistakenly identify themselves" (p. 228).

Helpers wrap themselves in their procedural authority, binding themselves so tightly in their concern for the right method, the latest technology, that it is no wonder that their actions then seem constricted. Helpers can never be seen as personal if they offer knowledge or skills instead of themselves. Murphy (1987) resented the trade: "What I needed was not a new instrument, but an old-fashioned clinician with plenty of intuition" (p. 14). Patients argue that their helpers routinely neglect their feelings, that they have bought the argument in favor of impersonality.

But whenever anyone mentions using either selves or intuitive traits therapeutically, practitioners stir uneasily. They have a problem with being intuitive or personal. Some actually call caring *feminine*. Lear (1980) claimed that her husband felt care from women, distance from men: "They were with him constantly, those woman figures. They were gentle and good. . . . The male figures were with him for ten minutes a day. They were marginal figures, shadowy and cold. They touched him with instruments—stethoscopes, blood-pressure gadgets" (pp. 40–41). It seems that here too helpers try to split the inseparable; they say that men will offer cures and skills, women service and caring. But patients argue that this and all other separations are unthinkable; all helpers must care.

Hodgins (1964) argued that encounters felt as personal are often what patients need most: "[The patient] will draw courage as he perceives human understanding underlying the professional techniques of those into whose care he has been given. Human understanding, however, is not to be found in the rituals of anything called medical science" (p. 841). Unhappily, concern for more personal issues seems to matter little in this formulaic belief: Correct procedures produce the superior results that serve the patient's best interests.

Occupational therapists are among those who must admit that techniques and protocols can preempt caring. Yerxa (1980) argued that "*technique*, once employed in the service of human needs, is rapidly moving us toward a society of total technology in which our ways of thinking and being themselves become so technical that we lose sight of other ways of thinking and being" (p. 530).

King (1980) concurred, claiming that "therapists have ignored their instinct for caring" (p. 525). Heller and Vogel (1986) described Heller's experience with the tight formula in his occupational therapy treatment for Guillain-Barré syndrome:

> As soon as I could sand a block of wood (with a need to rest both arms, it was written, after seven repetitions), a change was made to a coarser grade of sandpaper, increasing the amount of force required, and it was just as punishing for me to have to execute them as it had been in the beginning. (pp. 166–67)

Although Heller wanted to savor his gain and determine his next move in therapy, a protocol forbade his doing so.

Parham (1987) discussed the case of Longmore, a former faculty member at the University of Southern California Program in Disability and Society:

> He was subjected to long hours of occupational therapy training for self-care skills although he had no intention of performing these time-consuming tasks independently at home. He planned to hire an attendant who would expedite the process, freeing him to use his time and energy to pursue more stimulating and productive activities. (p. 556)

Neither Heller's nor Longmore's treatments heeded Baum's (1980) reminder that interventions notwithstanding, "we are nothing more than a bystander in the life of that individual until a relationship is formed" (p. 514).

A Health Care System Driven by Business, Efficiency, and Profit

Francis Peabody (1930), a physician, articulated the problem well when he argued that "hospitals, like other institutions, founded with the highest human ideals, are apt to deteriorate into dehumanized machines" (p. 33). Many narratives suggest that this dehumanization stems from a system of providing health care that builds on business, efficiency, and profit.

The business of health care. Any business that aims to offer individual service to large numbers of people may suffer from criticisms such as Sarton's (1988):

> A small incident at the hairdresser's has given me something to try to understand . . . While Donna was securing my hair into curlers, an old lady who was waiting to be picked up came and stood beside us and talked cheerfully about herself and her daughters and Donna responded. It was though I did not exist, was an animal being groomed. (p. 255)

The number of patients who seek treatment can compromise caring expressions in hospitals. As Sarason (1985) wrote, "The clinician becomes a rationer of time, and that obviously sets drastic limits on the degree to which the ever-present client need for caring and compassion can be met" (p. 170). The result of that rationing is the feeling articulated by Peter Peabody during his visits to a busy clinic: "I just feel like they don't give a damn. . . . I feel like I'm always being ignored, they don't care" (1986, p. 172). Additional complications associate with the business of hospitals, however, by virtue of their life-saving function. Hodgins (1964) discussed the personal estrangement that occurs with the rapid interventions warranted by life-threatening illness:

> Speaking as a patient, I think this point is important: that the stroke victim is most likely to encounter, as his first medical ministrant, a physician to whom he is a total stranger. Since speedy hospitalization is usually a first goal in stroke, treatment by strangers is likely to continue. (p. 839)

Peabody (1930) explained one consequence of the lifesaving business:

> When a patient enters a hospital, the first thing that commonly happens to him is that he loses his personal identity. He is generally referred to, not as Henry Jones, but as "that case of mitral stenosis in the second bed on the left". . . . It leads, more or less directly, to the patient being treated as a case of mitral stenosis, and not a sick man. (p. 31)

The problem is a matter of focus; the institutional eye sees the relevance of saving Henry's life and so does not capture the wider clinical picture—that although "Henry happens to have heart disease, he is not disturbed so much by dyspnea as he is by anxiety for the future" (Peabody, 1930, p. 34).

The efficiency of the health care system. Murphy (1987) has spoken to the kind of ordering that occurs in institutions, renaming the hospital an island invaded by a rationalized system of schedules and shifts: "The hospital has all the features of a bureaucracy, and, like bureaucracies everywhere, it both breeds and feeds on impersonality" (p. 21).

The impersonality is well illustrated in Saxton's (1987) account:

> The scariest part of the hospitalization for me was not the surgery but the doctor rounds. On the mornings when these rituals were scheduled, the nurses and aides awakened us much earlier than usual. Meals and wash-ups were rushed. . . . Then they would come, the surgeons, the residents, the interns. . . . They entered our ward, about fifteen adults. . . . Strange long words were uttered; bandages were opened and quickly closed. (p. 53)

Gebolys (1990) recalled that only on the fourth day of her hospital stay did a nurse's aide wash her hair, which was bloody and dirty from an automobile accident. The aide did so after her shift was over because the highly regulated day precluded this helping task. Sacks (1983) concluded that "the hospital, in short, is a singular mixture, where freedom and bondage, warmth and coldness, human and mechanical, life and death, are locked together in perpetual combat" (p. 24).

The battle sometimes seems insane, Murphy (1987) explained, because like most bureaucracies, the hospital has turned "capricious, arbitrary, and irresponsible as Wonderland's Red Queen" (p. 44). One feels the capriciousness in Beisser's (1989) experience with heartless caretakers:

> In one hospital, the first hour of the nurses' shift was spent in a detailed discussion of who would take coffee breaks when. Medications, patient needs, all other things paled in comparison. Sometimes people would literally leave you in midair in a lift to go on a coffee break, or leave you in some other awkward position, and just say, "It's my break time." (p. 35)

Brice (1987) recalled a nurse in the recovery room whom she asked for a blanket. The nurse, seeming much like the Red Queen, "barked 'I just brought you one; I'm not going to bring you another' and disappeared" (p. 31). People are a hospital's only possible conveyors of personal care; there can be no social life there if helpers are capricious and irresponsible. Sarton (1988) wearied of her treatment that was "bland at best, cold and inhuman at worst" (p. 103).

The profit of health care provision. Hodgins (1964) thought that helpers produce mostly problems with the profit-driven business of health care:

> We have heard much sentimental lamentation over the disappearance of the old "family physician"—dear, lovable old Dr. Peatmoss, who delivered all the babies, saw them through diphtheria, whooping cough and scarlet fever, sat at the deathbeds of the elderly, and never sent anyone a bill. This last lovable quality is, I suppose, why he disappeared. I felt no sense of personal loss at his passing because I never knew him. I should have liked to. The physicians in my life all had very efficient accounting systems—if not actual departments. (p. 840)

Longcope (1962), a physician, had argued even earlier that a business orientation causes "the 'quantification, mechanization and standardization' which are said to characterize this country" (p. 547). Within a business orientation to health care, knowledge takes coin value, cure becomes a high-priced commodity, and ill persons are transformed into buyers. Success and solvency turn into treatment goals, productivity and efficiency into the means to achieve them. In this scheme, more accrues from procedures that cure than from manners that care. Rabin (1982), a physician with amyotrophic lateral sclerosis, remembered that his physician gave him a pamphlet outlining the course of a disease that he already knew too well. He regretted that this physician gave him no suggestions about "how to muster the emotional strength to cope with a progressive degenerative disease" (p. 307).

Practitioners face a major quandary when their patients' needs for time and compassion compete with the institution's need to prosper. When high regard falls to those who treat the most patients or accumulate the most billable units of time, moments spent noticing, listening, or communicating are harder to justify. Sarason (1985) explained: "Whose agent I was became a pressing, daily, moral problem. I know what it is to have divided loyalties, to want to give up the fight, to rationalize away the internalized conflict" (pp. 170–171). And although few helpers buy the idea that patients are mere customers, many budget their caring actions. Patients experience the cuts as hurtful. Lear (1980) wrote of her husband's regret that he had never attended to his patients' experiences. He thought: "Damn it, doctors *should* know. They should care. Say how're they treating you? How's the food? Accommodations comfortable? Staff courteous? . . . . He himself would never even have thought to ask. Didn't that make him negligent too? Ah. Bingo" (p. 43).

Occupational Therapists Within the System

According to Sacks (1983), occupational therapists are among those who struggle more successfully against the impersonality within the health care provision system: "There are, of course, gaps in this totalitarian structure, where real care and affection still maintain a foothold; many of the 'lower' staff nurses, aides, orderlies, physiotherapists, speech therapists, etc. give themselves unstintingly, and with love, to their patients" (p. 24). But occupational therapists speak openly about the frustrations of clinical practice; as Howard (1991) wrote, "occupational therapy does not exist in a vacuum" (p. 878). Growing numbers of patients are a concern. Departments must handle more patients with fewer staff members because "productivity and efficiency are becoming high-priority goals" (p. 878). Howard argued that technological approaches are thus "valued more than the holistic use of a variety of methods" (p. 880).

The climate in hospitals seems one of "cost containment" rather than caring (Howard, 1991, p. 878). Kari and Michels (1991) wrote of their regret that "daily life for those living within the institution can become compartmentalized and focused on receiving services to alleviate dysfunction" (p. 721). Trahey (1991) saw the combat to which Sacks (1983) referred as a "struggle to integrate quality care with a businesslike approach to fiscal soundness" (p. 397). Burke and Cassidy (1991) called it the "disparity between reimbursement-driven practice and the humanistic values of occupational therapy" (p. 173). Boyle (1990) questioned one aspect of the dilemma:

> Are occupational therapists today meeting the needs of the rehabilitation population and considering their social, political, and economic status? Or are we compartmentalizing our services on the basis of our own need for neat, tidy treatment plans that fit our expertise and the selective mission of our institution? (p. 941)

940

The enormity of the challenge pressed Grady (1992) to ask a more fundamental question: "Is there still enjoyment in occupational therapy, or have we become so controlled with the realities of productivity, reimbursement, and modalities that we are failing to see the process as part of the outcome?" (p. 1063) A number of therapists have spoken to the powers essential for the struggle. Knowledge is one:

> All occupational therapists should have the knowledge, skills, and attitudes to position themselves to gain influence, power, and control of the systems in which they operate. To move upward in the power hierarchy, we must have knowledge (i.e., expertise), knowing (i.e., process skills), competencies, and credentials. (Nielson, 1991, p. 854)

But that competence, wrote Dickerson (1990), must be tempered by another concern: "Care must also be exercised so that therapists never sacrifice quality of care for increased profits" (p. 137).

The quality of care central to occupational therapy has traditionally included the assumption that "if therapists are to create individually designed, personally meaningful treatment programs, then they must spend considerable time and energy getting to know each patient as a person" (Burke & Cassidy, 1991, p. 173). More and more, according to Burke and Cassidy, occupational therapists "must use a technical, protocol-driven approach to treatment" (p. 174). "Like physicians," they wrote, "we have had to amend our traditional allegiance to the patient due to increased fiscal restraint, which requires that we now consider the economic realities of the hospitals in which we work" (p. 174).

Conclusion

Caregivers such as Vanderwoude (1988) have paused after the course of their own illness to explain: "My illness was beneficial in helping me to be more reflective, in teaching me an element of patience, and in heightening my understanding of the person facing possible terminal illness" (p. 125). Sacks (1984) was similarly convinced: "I saw that one must be a patient, and a patient among patients, that one must enter both the solitude and the community of patienthood, to have any idea of what 'being a patient' means" (p. 172). Although such an experience offers a profound form of knowing, first-person narratives can also inspire helpers to consider the manner in which they care.

Occupational therapists who choose how they will be among their patients do so within a context shaped by an intermingling of personal, professional, and societal beliefs. Occupational therapists have traditionally endorsed a practice based on competence and caring (Peloquin, 1990). Therapists who act as either technicians or authoritarian parents disappoint patients with their overvaluation of competence. Several societal beliefs can be seen to connect with such overly competent enactments:

an emphasis on the rational fixing of problems, an overreliance on method and protocol, and a health care system that thrives on business, efficiency, and profit.

A focus on fixing bodily parts and functional problems leads to a tendency to disregard a patient's understanding or feelings about illness. To a patient, the disregard feels technical rather than personal. A reliance on protocols that have success, authority, and reliability leads to a tendency to deny a patient's control, to dismiss a helper's intuition about what is right. To a patient, this preeminence of protocol feels impersonal and authoritarian. The routinization and rationalization of health care institutions lead to discourteous behaviors. The actions feel efficient but uncaring. Therapists who act as technicians or authoritarian parents reflect society's preference for the rational fixing of problems, the implementing of successful strategies, and the management of solvent businesses. And although each of these orientations is important and worthy of affirmation in any health care practice, overvaluation of any one of these can compromise the actions and words that mean care. Practice that values the person must build on both competence and caring.

Toward the end of his personal litany of complaints, Hodgins (1964) remembered the need that helpers also have for courage in the face of illness. He ended his address to the Academy of Physicians by suggesting that practitioners consider a picture of practice that might replenish their commitment: "Reclothe yourselves in humanity" (p. 843). It is hoped that occupational therapists will be among those who will hold fast to this image of personal caring as they practice competent care. ▲

Acknowledgment

The research on which this article is based constitutes a portion of a dissertation that partially fulfilled requirements for a doctoral degree conferred by the Institute for the Medical Humanities, the University of Texas Medical Branch, Galveston, Texas. The dissertation is entitled *Art in Practice: When Art Becomes Caring*.

References

Baum, C. M. (1980). Eleanor Clarke Slagle lecture — Occupational therapists put care in the health system. *American Journal of Occupational Therapy, 34,* 505–516.

Bailey, D. M. (1990). Reasons for attrition from occupational therapy. *American Journal of Occupational Therapy, 44,* 23–29.

Beisser, A. (1989). *Flying without wings: Personal reflections on becoming disabled.* New York: Doubleday.

Benziger, B. F. (1969). *The prison of my mind.* New York: Walker.

Boyle, M. A. (1990). The Issue Is — The changing face of the rehabilitation population: A challenge for therapists. *American Journal of Occupational Therapy, 44,* 941–945.

Brice, J. (1987). Empathy lost. *Harvard Medical Letter, 60,* 28–32.

Burke, J. P., & Cassidy, J. C. (1991). Disparity between reimbursement-driven practice and humanistic values of occupational therapy. *American Journal of Occupational Therapy*, *45*, 173–176.

Cassell, E. J. (1985). *Talking with patients: Volume 1. The theory of doctor–patient communication.* Cambridge: MIT Press.

Dickerson, A. (1990). Evaluating productivity and profitability in occupational therapy contractual work. *American Journal of Occupational Therapy*, *44*, 133–137.

Flagg, P. (1923). *The patient's viewpoint.* Milwaukee: Bruce Publishing.

Gebolys, E. (1990). Inadequacies, inequities and inanities in modern medicine—A personal experience. *Occupational Therapy Forum*, *12*, 6–7, 13–18.

Grady, A. P. (1992). Nationally Speaking—Occupation as vision. *American Journal of Occupational Therapy*, *46*, 1062–1065.

Heller, J., & Vogel, S. (1986). *No laughing matter.* New York: Avon.

Hodgins, E. (1964). Whatever became of the healing art? *Annals of the New York Academy of Sciences*, *164*, 838–846.

Howard, B. S. (1991). How high do we jump? The effect of reimbursement on occupational therapy. *American Journal of Occupational Therapy*, *45*, 875–881.

Jourard, S. (1964). *The transparent self: Self-disclosure and well being.* New York: Van Nostrand Reinhold.

Kari, N., & Michels, P. (1991). The Lazarus project: The politics of empowerment. *American Journal of Occupational Therapy*, *44*, 719–725.

King, L. J. (1980). Creative caring. *American Journal of Occupational Therapy*, *34*, 522–528.

Lear, M. (1980). *Heartsounds.* New York: Simon & Schuster.

Leder, D. (1984). Medicine and paradigms of embodiment. *Journal of Medicine and Philosophy*, *9*(1), 29–43.

Lee, L. (1987). Transcendence. In M. Saxton & F. Howe (Eds.), *With wings: An anthology of literature by and about women with disabilities* (pp. 109–116). New York: Feminist Press.

Longcope, W. (1962). Methods and medicine. In W. H. Davenport (Ed.), *The good physician: A treasury of medicine* (pp. 546–559). New York: Macmillan.

Mattingly, C. (1991). The narrative nature of clinical reasoning. *American Journal of Occupational Therapy*, *45*, 998–1005.

McClay, E. (1977). *Green winter: Celebrations of old age.* New York: Reader's Digest Press.

Moore, A. R. (1978). *The missing medical text: Humane patient care.* Melbourne, Australia: Melbourne University Press.

Murphy, R. F. (1987). *The body silent.* New York: Henry Holt.

Nielson, C. (1991). The Issue Is—Positioning for power. *American Journal of Occupational Therapy*, *45*, 853–854.

Parham, D. (1987). Nationally Speaking—Toward professionalism: The reflective therapist. *American Journal of Occupational Therapy*, *41*, 555–561.

Peabody, B. (1986). *The screaming room: A mother's journal of her son's struggle with AIDS.* New York: Avon.

Peabody, F. W. (1930). *Doctor and patient papers on the relationship of the physician to men and institutions.* New York: Macmillan.

Pekkanen, J. (1988). *M.D.: Doctors talk about themselves.* New York: Del Publishing.

Pellegrino, E. (1979). *Humanism and the physician.* Knoxville: University of Tennessee Press.

Peloquin, S. M. (1989). Sustaining the art of practice in occupational therapy. *American Journal of Occupational Therapy*, *43*, 219–226.

Peloquin, S. M. (1990). The patient–therapist relationship in occupational therapy: Understanding visions and images. *American Journal of Occupational Therapy*, *44*(1), 13–21.

Peloquin, S. M. (1993). The depersonalization of patients: A profile gleaned from narratives. *American Journal of Occupational Therapy*, *47*, 830–837.

Rabin, D., Rabin, P., & Rabin, R. (1982). Compounding the ordeal of ALS. *New England Journal of Medicine*, *307*, 506–509.

Reiser, D., & Schroder, A. K. (1980). *Patient interviewing: The human dimension.* Baltimore: Williams & Wilkins.

Sacks, O. (1983). *Awakenings.* New York: Dutton.

Sacks, O. (1984). *A leg to stand on.* New York: Harper & Row.

Sarason, S. B. (1985). *Caring and compassion in clinical practice.* San Francisco: Jossey-Bass.

Sarton, M. (1988). *After the stroke: A journal.* New York: Norton.

Saxton, M. (1987). In M. Saxton & F. Howe (Eds.), *With wings: An anthology of literature by and about women with disabilities* (pp. 51–57). New York: Feminist Press.

Schultz, S., & Schkade, J. K. (1992). Occupational adaptation: Toward a holistic approach for contemporary practice, Part 2. *American Journal of Occupational Therapy*, *46*, 917–925.

Taylor, R. (1972). *The practical art of medicine.* New York: Harper & Row.

Trahey, P. (1991). A comparison of the cost-effectiveness of two types of occupational therapy services. *American Journal of Occupational Therapy*, *45*, 397–400.

Van Eys, J. & McGovern, J. P., Eds. (1988). *The doctor as a person.* Illinois: Charles C Thomas.

Vanderwoude, J. (1988). The caregiver as a patient. In J. Van Eys & J. P. McGovern (Eds.), *The doctor as a person* (pp. 172–184). Illinois: Charles C Thomas.

Yerxa, E. J. (1980). Occupational therapy's role in creating a future climate of caring. *American Journal of Occupational Therapy*, *34*, 529–534.

THE ISSUE IS

Now That We Have Managed Care, Shall We Inspire It?

Suzanne M. Peloquin

Suzanne M. Peloquin, PhD, OTR, is Associate Professor, Department of Occupational Therapy, School of Allied Health Sciences, The University of Texas Medical Branch at Galveston, 301 University Boulevard, Galveston, Texas 77555-1028, and Consultant, Department of Occupational Therapy, Transitional Learning Community at Galveston, Galveston, Texas.

This article was accepted for publication December 24, 1995.

W e knew it, but Mary Foto said it: "Managed care 'is here to stay'" (as quoted by Hettinger, 1995, p. 19). It seems apt, then, that we come to terms with managed care—literally. And coming to terms is a process with which occupational therapists are familiar. Parham (1987) said that reflective practitioners name and frame their realities, using language and logic to first explain what they see (name) and then to spell out a course of action (frame). Although Parham discussed this process in the context of treatment, therapists might benefit from a reflection that names and frames managed care. This article aims to prompt such reflection while making this point: We have *managed* care, but we must continue to *inspire* it—to keep caring for the health of others central to our practice.

Before turning to this discussion, I will speak of my intent. Some readers may argue that an educator who is removed from clinical realities has no grounds for commenting on managed care. The argument has logic, but it does not consider that people can support one another from different vantage points. What therapists offer patients is an empathic but divergent perspective on their realities; we sometimes name it *hope*. This reflection has a similar aim. My purpose is to salute those who grapple with managed care and to offer suggestions that make sense from where I practice.

The Language and Logic of Managed Care

Some may argue that *managed care* is the ultimate oxymoron because it names an incongruence larger than *grateful dead*. More typically, descriptors of a different kind associate with the term *care*. Some descriptors name those who will receive care—child, elder, patient—and others name the type of care that will be given—critical, intensive, quality. The odd juxtaposition of managed care causes one to ask how management applies to care. Usually, a person is said to manage a budget or a household. Does care warrant such management?

Interestingly, the first dictionary definitions for management associate with the training and handling of horses. From these earlier meanings came the more familiar one of skillful handling, direction, or control (*Merriam-Webster's Collegiate Dictionary*, 1993). Given this understanding, one can better grasp the thinking of those who named managed care. A delivery system gone wild needed taming. Those who named the problem framed a congruent action. Unbridled excesses, runaway costs, and a galloping use of procedures invited management.

Syndicated columnist Dave Barry (1994) saw humor in the health care system's extravagance before managed care. He told the story of 8-year-old Natalie who modified a childrens' board game by putting the gamepieces in her nose. When one gamepiece accidentally went in the wrong direction during an intake breath, Natalie's parents took her to the hospital. Although the gamepiece was already in her digestive tract, the total bill was $3,200. Barry suggested that stool searches done at home are far cheaper.

Certainly, the cost of health care delivery needs to be managed, and a logical approach to managing cost is to control both access and use. Management extends beyond cost, however. As a business, health care delivery warrants accountability; as a human service, it needs ethical responsibility. Productivity, measurability of outcome, reasonableness of cost, efficiency of effort, quality of service, and justification of effectiveness are concepts fundamental to the practice of good business *and* ethical service. It is unfair to assume that the managed care industry has pressed practitioners toward functions that *oppose* good care.

Early in our profession's history, when a reconstruction aide named Ora Ruggles (Carlova & Ruggles, 1946) took leave from practice, Eleanor Clarke Slagle asked her to return, saying, "Get behind the effort and push!" (p. 113) Ruggles did so, starting occupational therapy departments in many places. More currently, Foto argued this need relative to managed care (Hettinger, 1995). Good management is an effort therapists can push. If over the years, occupational therapists failed to tend to good business, thus adding to the extravagance of health care delivery, they invited the redirection inherent in managed care. Therapists will always need to be good managers who are accountable for business and responsible for service, and in this context, managed care makes sense.

Managed Care: Naming the Incongruence

Boisaubin (1994) took a more serious look at runaway costs than Barry (1994) did, noting the larger implications of cost-containment:

> The Kaiser Permanente System found that it would save $3.5 million if it stopped using an expensive nonionic x-ray agent, even though the cheaper alternative caused more patient reactions. Most reactions have been mild and nonfatal; is it worth $3.5 million to avoid those reactions? However, in this tradeoff an occasional patient will encounter discomfort, morbidity, or even mortality. Ideally, the $3.5 million would be better spent on health screening to prevent 35 breast cancer deaths, 100 cervical cancer deaths, or 105 heart attacks. The once rhetorical debate focusing on the worth of a human life becomes all too realistic in this new calculus. (p. 1)

The management of extravagance is a powerful function; it can change the ways in which helpers offer care and patients receive it.

Occupational therapists have described the effects of managed care on their therapies. Noting the restrictions on access that have followed capitation, Kornblau (1995) asked:

> Is this legal? Yes. Health care is not a right. It is something agreed to in a contract between a coverage provider company and a policy purchaser.... Although the behavior is legal, I cannot help asking myself whether it is ethical. Is it right to give physicians monetary incentives to sacrifice care which would improve the quality of one's life? (p. 4).

Occupational therapists have described far-reaching outcomes of managed care, including shorter lengths of stay, cross

training, augmentation of revenues by raising patient volume, interdisciplinary treatment, fewer and shorter outpatient and home health services, and "one stop shopping" where patients can access many services in one place (Joe & Hettinger, 1995). Some therapists note that the managed care system has compromised care by turning it into a bureaucracy that forces poor treatment, misunderstanding of patient needs, disregard for therapists' opinions, delays in authorization, increased paperwork, and compromised reimbursement (Hettinger, 1995). Years before the introduction of the term *managed care,* many therapists cautioned against a growing press for productivity, efficiency, and profit that threatened humane practices (Baum, 1980; Boyle, 1990; Burke & Cassidy, 1991; Dickerson, 1990; Grady, 1992; Howard, 1991; Kari & Michels, 1991; Peloquin, 1993; Yerxa, 1980). The far-reaching controls of managed care, aimed first at excess, have limited care. How should therapists frame a response?

We might recall the appeals for reform of the health care system that invited a greater change than management. Many persons proposed a broader action with several aims, including universal access to adequate health care (Council on Ethical and Judicial Affairs, American Medical Association, 1995), comprehensive and affordable (quality) care by competent providers (Boisaubin, 1994), and a hope to focus on prevention and to personalize delivery (Boisaubin, 1994; Peloquin, 1993). This call to action transcends any response named *management.* Ron Anderson, a physician and administrator, said it well in his interview with PBS personality Bill Moyers (1993):

> You try to bring healing to a person and help them [sic] heal themselves. Many times, if they have information, and if they're empowered through a caring milieu, they will be better able to function. The doctors and nurses won't be going home with them, so it's very important that we get them to the highest plane of function that we can. We have a saying in our geriatric ward that we've never met a patient we couldn't care for. We've met many we couldn't cure. (p. 26)

Management—skillful handling, direction, and control—is a function of good care but only a part of good care. Even in the realm of horse training where the term *management* originated, trainers have suggested other actions:

> We shall have to give up our inclination to control our horse by force. Instead we shall have to try to learn to respect the way *he* wants to do things....And, instead of trying to impose on our particular animal our idea of what he should be able to achieve, we must first seek to learn what his capabilities really are...we shall have to add to our analytical capability an equal capacity for intuitive thought....Without this, our relationship with our horse will be one of spiritual warfare instead of harmony and beauty. (Hassler, 1994, p. 16)

In health care, when management issues preempt all other concerns, the ethos of caring and the art of practice are at risk.

There is much logic to the language of managed care, but that language seems inadequate to the task of caring. As Hayakawa (1969) noted, any one instrument has its limitations. A thermometer, made to read temperature, will not read color, weight, or odor. "Every language," said Hayakawa, "like the language of the thermometer, leaves work undone for other languages to do" (p. 8). Attention to sound management principles, one valid approach to reforming health care delivery, leaves work undone; it needs to be part of a larger vision and responsivity.

Naming and Framing Another Response

In his reflections about education, Davies (1991) said much that may help this discussion. From his position on a state governing board, Davies concluded that the regulatory function of those on state boards is mere background; their essential function is to inspire education. A question that he thought board members must ask is this: "Are we helping to create an environment in which teaching and learning are honored and can flourish?" (p. 58). He said that the making of that environment is a call to (a) engender a restlessness throughout the system, (b) disturb complacency, and (c) insist that rules be broken when there is good and sufficient reason.

The health care system invites a similar effort. Occupational therapists must see their business functions as a vital background to good practice. Because they have high stakes in health care delivery, therapists *must* manage themselves well. They must get behind the management effort. But they must also ask whether they are making an environment that nourishes care for the health of others. They might then name and frame a more essential action: inspire care.

Why should occupational therapists inspire health care delivery? To *inspire* is to exert a livening influence, to animate or hearten the spirit (*Merriam-Webster's Collegiate Dictionary*, 1993). To inspire is to make something happen—to build something—from the inside out. Inspiration is a form of edification. The various systems within which therapists practice need inspiration if they will emerge reformed. And occupational therapists are immersed in the kind of making that inspires.

Since its origins, occupational therapy has made inspiration a basic function. The strong link between occupation and the human spirit is well-portrayed by Petersen (1976):

> There is a shouting SPIRIT
> deep inside me:
> TAKE CLAY, it cries,
> TAKE PEN AND INK,
> TAKE FLOUR AND WATER,
> TAKE A SCRUB BRUSH,
> TAKE A YELLOW CRAYON,
> TAKE ANOTHER'S HAND—
> AND WITH ALL THESE SAY YOU,
> SAY LOVING.
> So much of who I am
> is subtly spoken
> in my making. (p. 61)

Meaningful occupation, the core of our therapy, animates and extends the human spirit.

The founders of the profession often spoke of its spiritual aims. Barton (1920) named occupational therapy a *making*—not of a product, but of a person stronger physically, mentally, and

spiritually than before. The inspiring action of occupational therapy is well-described by Ruggles (Carlova & Ruggles, 1946): "It is not enough to give a patient something to do with his hands. You must reach for the heart as well as the hands. It's the heart that really does the healing" (p. 69).

On a systemic level, occupational therapists are also animators. Whether they practice in hospitals or schools, prisons or community programs, therapists hear comments that note their singularity in livening the settings within which they work. Occupational therapy clinics are alive; therapists make life worlds that inspire and empower.

Inspiration is a function of occupational therapy; it is familiar and basic. It seems fitting that we stand among those who manage responsibly while also inspiring care for the health of others.

Inspiring Care: Moving Past the Rhetoric

The features of managed care—efficiency, accountability, and cost containment—have become familiar, and we recognize in them the actions of good business. But how shall we recognize the actions that inspire care? As long as they shape an environment in which caring for the health of others is central, these actions may take many forms. And whether this shaping occurs on a large or small scale, its function might, as Davies (1991) suggested, engender a restlessness throughout the system, disturb complacency, and cause any rules that compromise health care to be broken with good reason.

Therapists might consider the following example a large action aimed at the rules of managed care. *OT Week* ran part of an article from *The Washington Post* about the bills spearheaded by physicians and passed by five legislatures (Doctors Take on Managed Care, 1995). These bills restricted managed care business practices "in the name of patient protection" (p. 12). The Arkansas law, for example, requires that every health maintenance organization

(HMO) allow patients to see any physician who will accept the HMO rate, thereby increasing access. Occupational therapists can launch like efforts. At the very least, they can lend support to those who inspire the system politically.

Therapists might consider the following to be an action that challenges the rules but on a smaller scale. Many persons spend time writing letters to justify treatment or advocate therapy; the letters propose a broader view of health. Whenever caring for a person's health becomes more central to payers as a result of these letters, the therapists who wrote them can claim to have inspired health care.

As I considered the smaller actions that inspire, I saw a woman walking briskly down my street. Although walkers are common in my neighborhood, she caught my attention because she carried a brown bag and moved from one side of the road to the other, grabbing up curbside litter. I was inspired. Nested within her personal routine (exercise) was an action that launched a larger effort (neighborhood cleanup).

Persons can inspire most of the systems within which they function. In 2 to 3 minutes, sales cashiers can liven someone's day. If a form of inspiration can occur within such short time frames, there is cause to believe that therapists can, over longer periods, make caring for health a more central concern among patients, coworkers, administrators, and third-party payers.

One of our founders named the inspiration that can edify our practice as he spoke to a group of graduating students:

> May you realize in increasing measure the value of certain spiritual things which are the real making of life, but which we call by many common names. Kindness, humanity, decency, honor, good faith—to give these up under any circumstances whatever would be a loss greater than any defeat, or even death itself. (Kidner, 1929, p. 385)

The call to manage *and* inspire care is a plea to bring to life forms of health care delivery that manage the system and animate the act of caring about health.

Actions That Inspire: A Sampling

The following are general suggestions for inspiring the health care delivery system. Each has a background managerial function within which nests a more essential and inspiring function (B. C. Abreu, personal communication, October 15, 1995). These suggestions make sense within the context of this reflection, and they seem sound to clinicians with whom I have shared them. Admittedly, they lack the particularity of application that persons who enact them might provide. I offer them to those who seek possibilities.

1. Infuse competent treatment with kindness, decency, honor, and good faith.
   Managerial function. This action makes a good "package deal" for patients, payers, and referral sources.
   Inspirational function. We do the right thing for our clients.

2. Introduce, research, and publicize clinical improvements, flexible approaches, and creative managing techniques.
   Managerial function. This action establishes our efficacy as therapists, our artistry as practitioners, and our skill as managers.
   Inspirational function. We promote practice by showing what we do and telling how it works.

3. Include in clinical pathways and practice guidelines the protocols and critical outcomes that address physical and mental health in the broad sense.
   Managerial function. This measure is cost-effective in the long run.
   Inspirational function. We retain our holistic heritage.

4. Speak with logic and passion for patients whose health depends on longer stays and more therapy.
   Managerial function. This action reclaims consumers at risk and offers good service.

Inspirational function. We temper limited access with strong advocacy.

5. Educate clients with a knowledge that leads them to prevent dysfunction and manage themselves.
   Managerial function. This action taps a new market and supports a goal of managed care.
   Inspirational function. We enact our ethos of helping others to help themselves.

6. Declare boldly and widely (at local, state, and national levels) the links between human occupation and health.
   Managerial function. This action touts our unique position in health care systems.
   Inspirational function. We promote the profession's core function, values, and standards.

7. Open channels that foster dialogue with managed care personnel.
   Managerial function. This action affirms our worth as players in the system.
   Inspirational function. We declare aims for reform broader than cost containment.

8. Assume leadership roles (e.g., members of quality improvement councils, case managers, case reviewers) in the systems within which we practice.
   Managerial function. This action shows systems personnel that we are savvy leaders.
   Inspirational function. We take positions from which to argue a vision of health that includes occupation.

9. Monitor and support larger political actions (e.g., legislation, coalitions).
   Managerial function. This action helps us shape policy.
   Inspirational function. We press for health care delivery that is managed, caring, and ethical.

10. Apply sound problem-solving approaches to paperwork and business tasks.

Managerial function. This action jostles the sluggishness of reimbursement.
   Inspirational function. We make more time for caring.

11. Cultivate among practitioners a respect for business principles.
   Managerial function. This action supports quality-process models (i.e., total quality management, continuous quality improvement).
   Inspirational function. We include in process monitoring the actions that meet high standards.

12. Collaborate with those whose vision (i.e., caring for the health of others) supports our own.
   Managerial function. This action gains us strength in numbers and conveys our faith in teams.
   Inspirational function. We cause deeper and better reform.

When Hall (1922) spoke about the task faced by the Society for the Promotion of Occupational Therapy, he could have been noting the challenge we face today: "It seems reasonable to assert that here is a work of national importance, a human reclamation service touching vitally on matters of vast social and economic consequence" (p. 164). We have begun to manage health care delivery, and there is logic in our getting behind that effort. But we can reclaim more.

Health care reform is a building from the inside that calls for a greater responsivity than any form of management that shapes from the outside in. Health care reform, in its truest sense, is an edification through actions large and small—it is the making of an environment in which caring for the health of others is central. When it comes to health care delivery, the issue goes past the logic that we must manage care to this question: Shall we inspire it? ▲

References

Barry, D. (1994). *The world according to Dave Barry*. New York: Wing.

Barton, G. E. (1920). What occupational therapy may mean to nursing. *Trained Nurse and Hospital Review, 64,* 304–310.

Baum, C. M. (1980). Eleanor Clarke Slagle lecture—Occupational therapists put care in the health system. *American Journal of Occupational Therapy, 34,* 505–516.

Boisaubin, E. V. (1994, May). Ethical and legal dilemmas in managed care. *Medical Humanities Rounds, 11,* 1–2.

Boyle, M. A. (1990). The Issue Is— The changing face of the rehabilitation population: A challenge for therapists. *American Journal of Occupational Therapy, 44,* 941–945.

Burke, J. P., & Cassidy, J. C. (1991). The Issue Is—Disparity between reimbursement driven practice and humanistic values of occupational therapy. *American Journal of Occupational Therapy, 45,* 173–176.

Carlova, J., & Ruggles, O. (1946). *The healing heart.* New York: Julian Messner.

Council on Ethical and Judicial Affairs, American Medical Association. (1995). Ethical issues in managed care. *Journal of the American Medical Association, 273,* 331–335.

Davies, G. K. (1991). Teaching and learning: What are the questions? *Teaching Education, 4*(1), 57–61.

Dickerson, A. (1990). Evaluating pro- ductivity and profitability in occupational therapy contractual work. *American Journal of Occupational Therapy, 44,* 133–137.

Doctors take on managed care. (1995, September 14). *OT Week, 9*(37), 12.

Grady, A. P. (1992). Nationally Speaking—Occupation as vision. *American Journal of Occupational Therapy, 46,* 1062–1065.

Hall, H. J. (1922). Editorial—American Occupational Therapy Association. *Archives of Occupational Therapy, 1,* 163–165.

Hassler, J. K. (1994). *Beyond the mirror—The study of the mental and spiritual aspects of horsemanship.* Quarryville, PA: Goals Unlimited.

Hayakawa, S. I. (1969). Introduction. In Gyorgy Kepes, *Language of vision* (pp. 1–11). Chicago: Paul Theobald.

Hettinger, J. (1995, September 7). Hand therapy in the grip of managed care. *OT Week, 9*(36), 18–20.

Howard, B. S. (1991). How high do we jump? The effect of reimbursement on occupational therapy. *American Journal of Occupational Therapy, 45,* 875–881.

Joe, B., & Hettinger, J. (1995, July 27). Hand therapy in the grip of managed care. *OT Week, 9*(30), 18–20.

Kari, N., & Michels, P. (1991). The Lazarus Project: The politics of empowerment. *American Journal of Occupational Therapy, 44,* 719–725.

Kidner, T. B. (1929). Address to graduates. *Occupational Therapy and Rehabilitation, 8,* 379–385.

Kornblau, B. (1995, July 31). Capitation could kill commitment. *Advance for Occupational Therapists,* 4.

Merriam-Webster's collegiate dictionary (10th ed.). (1993). Springfield, MA: Merriam-Webster.

Moyers, B. (1993). *Healing and the mind.* New York: Doubleday.

Parham, D. (1987). Nationally Speaking—Toward professionalism: The reflective therapist. *American Journal of Occupational Therapy, 41,* 555–561.

Peloquin, S. M. (1993). The patient–therapist relationship: Beliefs that shape care. *American Journal of Occupational Therapy, 47,* 935–942.

Petersen, J. (1976). *A book of yes.* Niles, IL: Argus.

Yerxa, E. J. (1980). Occupational therapy's role in creating a future climate of caring. *American Journal of Occupational Therapy, 34,* 529–534.

Brute

You must never again set your anger upon a patient. You were tired, you said, and therefore it happened. Now that you have excused yourself, there is no need for me to do it for you.

Imagine that you yourself go to a doctor because you have chest pain. You are worried that there is something the matter with your heart. Chest pain is your Chief Complaint. It happens that your doctor has been awake all night with a patient who has been bleeding from a peptic ulcer of his stomach. He is tired. That is your doctor's Chief Complaint. I have chest pain, you tell him. I am tired, he says.

Still I confess to some sympathy for you. I know what tired is.

Listen: It is twenty-five years ago in the Emergency Room. It is two o'clock in the morning. There has been a day and night of stabbings, heart attacks and automobile accidents. A commotion at the door: A huge black man is escorted by four policemen into the Emergency Room. He is handcuffed. At the door, the man rears as though to shake off the men who cling to his arms and press him from the rear. Across the full length of his forehead is a laceration. It is deep to the bone. I know it even without proving its depths. The split in his black flesh is like the white wound of an ax in the trunk of a tree. Again and again he throws his head and shoulders forward, then back, rearing, roaring. The policemen ride him like parasites. Had he horns he would gore them. Blind and trussed, the man shakes them about, rattles them. But if one of them loses his grip, the others are still fixed and sucking. The man is hugely drunk—toxic, fuming, murderous—a great mythic beast broken loose in the city, surprised in his night raid by a phalanx of legionnaires armed with clubs and revolvers.

I do not know the blow that struck him on the brow. Or was there any blow? Here is a brow that might have burst on its own, spilling out its excess rage, bleeding itself toward ease. Perhaps it was done by a jealous lover, a woman, or a man who will not pay him the ten dollars he won on a bet, or still another who has hurled the one insult that he cannot bear to hear. Perhaps it was done by the police themselves. From the distance of many years and from the safety of my little study, I choose to see it thus:

The helmeted corps rounds the street corner. A shout. "There he is!" And they clatter toward him. He stands there for a moment, lurching. Something upon which he had been feeding falls from his open mouth. He turns to face the policemen. For him it is not a new challenge. He is scarred as a Zulu from his many battles. Almost from habit he ascends to the combat. One or more of them falls under his flailing arms until—there is the swing of a truncheon, a sound as though a melon has been dropped from a great height. The white wedge appears upon the sweating brow of the black man, a waving fall of blood pours across his eyes and cheeks.

The man is blinded by it; he is stunned. Still he reaches forth to make contact with the enemy, to do one more piece of damage. More blows to the back, the chest and again to the face. Bloody spume flies from his head as though lifted by a great wind. The police are spattered with it. They stare at each other with an abstract horror and disgust. One last blow, and, blind as Samson, the black man undulates, rolling in a splayfooted circle. But he does not go down. The police are upon him then, pinning him, cuffing his wrists, kneeing him toward the van. Through the back window of the wagon—a netted panther.

In the Emergency Room he is led to the treatment area and to me. There is a vast dignity about him. He keeps his own counsel. What is he thinking? I wonder. The police urge him up on the table. They put him down. They restrain his arms with straps. I examine the wound, and my heart sinks. It is twelve centimeters long, irregular, jagged and, as I knew, to the skull. It will take at least two hours.

I am tired. Also to the bone. But something else . . . Oh, let me not deny it. I am ravished by the sight of him, the raw, untreated flesh, his very wildness which suggests less a human than a great and beautiful animal. As though by the addition of the wound, his body is more than it was, more of a body. I begin to cleanse and debride the wound. At my touch, he stirs and groans. "Lie still," I tell him. But now he rolls his head from side to side so that I cannot work. Again and again he lifts his pelvis from the table, strains against his bonds, then falls heavily. He roars something, not quite language. "Hold still," I say. "I cannot stitch your forehead unless you hold still."

Perhaps it is the petulance in my voice that makes him resume his struggle against all odds to be free. Perhaps he understands that it is only a cold, thin official voice such as mine, and not the billy clubs of half-a-dozen cops that can rob him of his dignity. And so he strains and screams. But why can he not sense that I am tired? He spits and curses and rolls his head to escape from my fingers. It is quarter to three in the morning. I have not yet begun to stitch. I lean close to him; his steam fills my nostrils. "Hold still," I say.

"*You* fuckin' hold still," he says to me in a clear, fierce voice. Suddenly, I am in the fury with him. Somehow he has managed to capture me, to pull me inside his cage. Now we are two brutes hissing and batting at each other. But I do not fight fairly.

I go to the cupboard and get from it two packets of heavy, braided silk suture and a large curved needle. I pass one of the heavy silk sutures through the eye of the needle. I take the needle in the jaws of a needle holder, and I pass the needle through the center of his right earlobe. Then I pass the needle through the mattress of the stretcher. And I tie the thread tightly so that his head is pulled to the right. I do exactly the same to his left earlobe, and again I tie the thread tightly so that his head is facing directly upward.

"I have sewn your ears to the stretcher," I say. "Move, and you'll rip 'em off." And leaning close I say in a whisper, "Now *you* fuckin' hold still."

I do more. I wipe the gelatinous clots from his eyes so that he can see. And I lean over him from the head of the table, so that my face is directly above his, upside down. And I grin. It is the cruelest grin of my life. Torturers must grin like that, beheaders and operators of racks.

But now he does hold still. Surely it is not just fear of tearing his earlobes. He is too deep into his passion for that. It is more likely some beastly wisdom that tells him that at last he has no hope of winning. That it is time to cut his losses, to slink off into high grass. Or is it some sober thought that pierces his wild brain, lacerating him in such a way that a hundred nightsticks could not? The thought of a woman who is waiting for him, perhaps? Or a child who, the next day and the week after that, will stare up at his terrible scars with a silent wonder that will shame him? For whatever reason, he is perfectly still.

It is four o'clock in the morning as I take the first stitch in his wound. At five-thirty, I snip each of the silks in his earlobes. He is released from his leg restrainers and pulled to a sitting position. The bandage on his head is a white turban. A single drop of blood in each earlobe, like a ruby. He is a maharajah.

The police return. All this time they have been drinking coffee with the nurses, the orderlies, other policemen, whomever. For over three hours the man and I have been alone in our devotion to the wound. "I have finished," I tell them. Roughly, they haul him from the stretcher and prod him toward the door. "Easy, easy," I call after them. And, to myself, if you hit him again . . .

Even now, so many years later, this ancient rage of mine returns to peck among my dreams. I have only to close my eyes to see him again wielding his head and jaws, to hear once more those words at which the whole of his trussed body came hurtling toward me. How sorry I will always be. Not being able to make it up to him for that grin.

The Hen Who Wouldn't Fly

Source: *Fables for Our Time*. Copyright 1940 by James Thurber. Reprinted by arrangement with Rosemary A. Thurber and The Barbara Hogenson Agency.

In one of the Midwestern states there lived a speckled hen who was opposed to aviation. In her youth, watching a flight of wild geese going north, she had seen two fall (shot by hunters), go into a nose dive, and crash into the woods. So she went about the countryside saying that flying was very dangerous and that any fowl with any sense would stick to the solid earth. Every time she had to cross a concrete highway near her farm she ran on foot, screaming and squawking; sometimes she made it easily, at other times she was almost tagged by passing cars. Five of her sisters and three of her daughters' husbands were killed trying to cross the road in one month (July).

Before long an enterprising wood duck set up an airways service across the road and back. He charge five grains of corn to take a hen or a rooster across, two grains for a chick. But the speckled hen, who was a power in the community, went around clucking and cut-cutting and cadawcutting and telling everybody that air travel was not safe and never would be. She persuaded the chickens not to ride on the duck's back, and he failed in business and returned to the forests. Before the year was out, the speckled hen, four more of her sisters, three of her sons-in-law, four aunts, and a grandfather had been killed trying to cross the road on foot.

Moral: Use the wings God gave you, or nothing can save you.

The Scotty Who Knew Too Much

Source: *Fables for Our Time*. Copyright 1940 by James Thurber. Reprinted by arrangement with Rosemary A. Thurber and The Barbara Hogenson Agency.

Several summers ago there was a Scotty who went to the country for a visit. He decided that all the farm dogs were cowards, because they were afraid of a certain animal that had a white stripe down its back. "You are a pussy-cat and I can lick you," the Scotty said to the farm dog who lived in the house where the Scotty was visiting. "I can lick the little animal with the white strip, too. Show him to me." "Don't you want to ask any questions about him?" said the farm dog. "Naw," said the Scotty. "*You* ask the questions."

So the farm dog took the Scotty into the woods and showed him the white-striped animal and the Scotty closed in on him, growling and slashing. It was all over in a moment and the Scotty lay on his back. When he came to, the farm dog said, "What happened?" "He threw vitriol," said the Scotty, "but he never laid a glove on me."

A few days later the farm dog told the Scotty there was another animal all the farm dogs were afraid of. "Lead me to him," said the Scotty. "I can lick anything that doesn't wear horseshoes." "Don't you want to ask any questions about him?" said the farm dog. "Naw," said the Scotty. "Just show me where he hangs out." So the farm dog led him to a place in the woods and pointed out the little animal when he came along. "A clown," said the Scotty, "a pushover," and he closed in, leading with his left and exhibiting some mighty fancy footwork. In less than a second the Scotty was flat on his back, and when he woke up the farm dog was pulling quills out of him. "What happened?" said the farm dog. "He pulled a knife on me," said the Scotty, "but at least I have learned how you fight out here in the country, and now I am going to beat *you* up." So he closed in on the farm dog, holding his nose with one front paw to ward off the vitriol and covering his eyes with the other front paw to keep out the knives. The Scotty couldn't see his opponent and he couldn't smell his opponent and he was so badly beaten that he had to be taken back to the city and put in a nursing home.

Moral: It is better to ask some of the questions than to know all the answers.

The Very Proper Gander

Not so very long ago there was a very fine gander. He was strong and smooth and beautiful and he spent most of his time singing to his wife and children. One day somebody who saw him strutting up and down in his yard and singing remarked, "There is a very proper gander." An old hen overheard this and told her husband about it that night in the roost. "They said something about propaganda," she said. "I have always suspected that," said the rooster, and he went around the barnyard next day telling everybody that the very fine gander was a dangerous bird, more than likely a hawk in gander's clothing. A small brown hen remembered a time when at a great distance she had seen the gander talking with some hawks in the forest. "They were up to no good," she said. A duck remembered that the gander had once told him he did not believe in anything. "He said to hell with the flag, too," said the duck. A guinea hen recalled that she had once seen somebody who looked very much like the gander throw something that looked a great deal like a bomb. Finally everybody snatched up sticks and stones and descended on the gander's house. He was strutting in his front yard, singing to his children and his wife. "There he is!" everybody cried. "Hawk-lover! Unbeliever! Flag-hater! Bomb-thrower!" So they set upon him and drove him out of the country.

Moral: Anybody who you or your wife thinks is going to overthrow the government by violence must be driven out of the country.

The Fairly Intelligent Fly

A Large spider in an old house built a beautiful web in which to catch flies. Every time a fly landed on the web and was entangled in it the spider devoured him, so that when another fly came along he would think the web was a safe and quiet place in which to rest. One day a fairly intelligent fly buzzed around above the web so long without lighting that the spider appeared and said, "Come on down." But the fly was too clever for him and said, "I never light where I don't see other flies and I don't see any other flies in your house." So he flew away until he came to a place where there were a great many other flies. He was about to settle down among them when a bee buzzed up and said, "Hold it, stupid, that's flypaper. All those flies are trapped." "Don't be silly," said the fly, "they're dancing." So he settled down and became stuck to the flypaper with all the other flies.

Moral: There is no safety in numbers, or in anything else.

Pinch

From Oates, Joyce Carol. *The Assignation.* New York: Ecco Press). Copyright 1988 by The Ontario Review, Inc. First published by The Ecco Press in 1988. Reprinted by permission of The Ecco Press.

She must have swallowed a tiny pit, or a thorn, that made its way into the fatty tissue of her left breast and would not budge. Day after day, during the night, stealthily, she felt it there—pinching the flesh until it ached.

She made her way to the radiology department of the hospital, bearing a green slip. A young nurse led her to the women's gowning room which had a close, tropical smell. There, she undressed quickly with a fear that someone would interrupt her. She put on a green smock, many times too large for her, open at the back, that tied at the nape of the neck but flapped open as she walked.

Led by the nurse to the X-ray room she saw how, in the corridor, many eyes followed her.

The X-ray room was windowless and air-conditioned. In it, a single mammoth machine rose to the ceiling. She stood staring at it as the nurse helped her disrobe, her breasts like drooping melons, sallow and blue-veined. The nipples looked worn, cracked, as if they had been sucked and gnawed numberless times, which was not the case. "You may find the machine cold at first," the nurse said. It was a warning couched in kindness. "It may pinch a little."

Though she was a tall woman she stood on a stool so that the nurse could fit her breast into the clamp. It had to be held tight, slightly flattened; the nurse had difficulty adjusting it and had to try several times. She told the woman to lean forward, no, to learn forward and to the side, like this, as if she were resting, relaxed, her armpit snug against a bar. The bar was cold. The clamp hurt her breast. "It may pinch a little," the nurse said again, tightening the clamp so that the woman bit her lip but did not cry out as she believed she was expected to do.

The nurse hid herself adroitly behind a shield. A sudden whirring noise filled the room as the machine came to life and the woman stood on the stool with her eyes closed.

"Now, the other side," said the nurse brightly.

The breast was unclamped and the other breast inserted. Again the woman leaned forward and to the side, trying to relax, her armpit pressed against a bar. The procedure was done twice over and when it was finished the nurse left the room with the X-ray film and the woman was allowed to sit, weak, shivering, at the end of an examining table with stirrups. Both her breasts were sore and she imagined that her left nipple had begun to bleed but she did not examine it closely. She had been told to put the green smock back on; with unsteady fingers she tied the strings at the nape of her neck.

After forty minutes a doctor came to examine her. The nurse returned with the X-ray photographs which he examined for some time, frowning. The doctor was a short, dapper, nearly bald man: a stranger: the woman had never seen him before and avoided his eyes now. She was told his name but did not hear it.

He asked her to disrobe and she did so, but slowly. The doctor's fingers were skillful and deft but her breasts were already sore from the machine and as he prodded and squeezed and manipulated and flattened her flesh the woman bit her lip to keep from crying out. The doctor then asked her to lie back on the examining table, which she did, though slowly, as if the request were an unnatural one. Tears ran out of the corners of the woman's eyes when her head came to rest on the flat leather pillow.

Now the doctor stands over her kneading her breasts vigorously. He stands with his head inclined as if he is listening for something the woman can't hear. He asks her questions, her voice replies intelligently, but in a neutral tone, as if from a distance. She might be speaking over the telephone. She is not crying now and there is really no evidence that she has been crying, if she has been crying.

The doctor has gone away, the woman and the nurse are left alone together in the X-ray room. It has become difficult for the woman to hear voices over the hum of the air conditioning but she understands that more X-rays are required and she intends to obey. She sees for the first time that the nurse is quite pretty, with a plump flushed face, plump reddened lips. The nurse helps her step up onto the stool, and helps fit her breast into the clamp. "This may pinch a little," the nurse says, licking her pretty lips.

Art in Practice: When Art Becomes Caring

Suzanne Marie Peloquin, MA, OTR, dissertation presented to the faculty of the University of Texas Graduate School of Biomedical Sciences at Galveston in partial fulfillment of the requirements for the degree of Doctor of Philosophy, the University of Texas Medical Branch at Galveston, December, 1991.

Works That Act to Enhance Empathy

One primary complaint from patients is that their helpers do not seem to grasp on the level of feeling that illness deeply disrupts their lives. Works of art can move a practitioner closer to an understanding of this frightening disruption. The evocative power of art can awaken a sense of what it is like to be ill. One rousing work is the painting *Burned Face* by the Dutch artist Karel Appel. Completed in 1961 in the style called Action Painting, the picture is marked by the bold colors and vigorous brush strokes that characterize this particular form of Abstract Expressionism. The painting is large, about ten feet high and seven feet wide. The right third of the painting is occupied mostly by shades of orange and a pinkish-beige, the orange filling the bottom half and running into beige only toward the top. The left third consists mostly of a black and a bluish-purple layered onto an orange that sometimes seeps through the darkness. The middle third holds more blues and blacks applied mostly in ragged patches but sometimes in slashes or strings. Brushed into these are dobs and squiggles of orange and flesh, smears and smudges of red. The pigments look thick in places and often run into one another, crawling and zigzagging, mixing and feathering across the canvas. Many of the strokes look random and careless.

The title of the painting, *Burned Face*, forces one to see that this is a picture of a person. The patches and dobs of flesh-colored pigment that can be seen as skin, the hint of two nostrils positioned as they would be on a face, and the ragged outline of a head rising from a blackened neck affirm, on closer look, that this is a person whose face is horribly burned and looking out at the viewer from a hot-orange background. When people see this painting without the benefit of its title, do they see a person's face? Perhaps. I did not. I first saw brambles and thorns, flowers growing and blossoming in a windswept desert. Until I saw the title, I failed to see any hint of face.

Because it is designed to share powerful truths about the reality of being so burned, this painting can enhance my awareness of another. The artist asks that I consider what it must be *like* to be so horrible burned, to take the perspective of one so damaged. The colors tell of the physical pain. I feel the searing heat both at this person's back and in the bubbling beneath the blacks and blues of this pained face. The smears and smudges of black and flesh show the charred skin of features burned away; slashing reds suggest blood that seeps from open wounds. The painting's title tells of a burning that happened in the past, but the colors and their application show a burning that continues. And with such an injury, the burning flares in treatments that strip off pieces of dead skin, that scissor-trim too close to newly-grown nerves, that press ointments into and wrap gauze around a soreness that seems forever. Throughout, there is a struggle to keep a balance of vital fluids, because, as in this painting, these rush to escape the body without its protection of skin. Even though they are not the true colors of burns, the blacks and blues in Kappel's work seem true to the never-ending pain.

A different kind of pain arrives as scar tissue forms. The squiggles and rough-edged patches on this canvas suggest the itch and crawl of slow healing. The textured blobs of orange and flesh foretell the ruddy scars that will fade only in time. Scars are thick; the skin once scarred will not be the same, never breathing as it did, never sweating as it did. Easy exchange with the surrounding air will not happen again. When skin grafts are used to remake the face, these will be small and patchy, like the smears and smudges of this painting; pieces of thigh taken to make cheeks, leg-skin not quite sure how to behave as a face. The melanin, too, is assaulted in a burn, and new skin may never match the old; the motley face in this painting is a color version of the disruption. Only pressure masks worn day and night will contain the furious growth such as that painted by Appel. And even after the raging of the burn and its awful treatment, will the fire not live on in its scars?

If one has such a burn, does looking in the mirror or glancing in a store-window cause real doubt about whether one has a face at all? Ugly seams and lumpy blotches replace the once-familiar freckle, the curve and color of lip, the chicken pox scar, all landmarks that spoke quietly but reassuringly of a once-familiar self. Gone forever are the old ways of pursing the lips, of wrinkling the brow, of closing the eyes. When the face and its many expressions are gone, does the self go into hiding?

I am forced to ask whether a face is something I have, or an essential component of who I am. Surely my face is who I am. Without a face to reflect my feelings, could I make my meanings known to others? Without a face, could I ask others to meet and return my gaze? Might I wonder if somewhere under all of this burned flesh my face and I lived on, the same as before only trapped behind this hideous mask? Or might I understand that I had in some awful moment turned into ropey flesh? I would lose a large measure of what I know to be me if I were to lose my face tomorrow. And so it must be for a patient so burned.

Often on the day-to-day, individuals discuss their dealings with the world in metaphorical terms that recall the face. People say, "I don't think I can face another day of this." Does this become the common parlance of one so burned? This painting communicates the despair; eyes that only yesterday opened to face challenges or closed to escape threats, disappear in the chaos of this burning. Looking out at the rest of the world seems impossible. Does each new day for one so burned bring the horror of not-facing the world? Most people encourage one another through their difficult times, saying "Keep your chin up," or "Keep a stiff upper lip." Does a person so horribly burned take only pain from metaphors that recall a face that is gone? Friends promise that time is a healer, but time will only scar a face that is burned.

For those who look upon this face can there be more than horror? When individuals look at persons in the world to know them, they grasp essential features. If they understand a face as eyes and eyebrows, nose and cheeks, mouth and teeth, then a burned face is not a face at all, and they will be appalled by claims to a likeness that is not there. How much acceptance follows bodily wholeness? Is fellowship only skin-deep? When does the shunning of turning heads and whispering voices begin? When a finger is obliterated? An arm? An ear? A nose? And if one dares, instead of shunning, to make a connection with one so burned, where should one

look? Appel knows the dilemma; he hides the eyes. Looking into this face will be hard. Direct eye contact will be awkward, a loving gaze impossible. This face is ugly by all the standards of facial beauty. Who among friends and family members will not cringe? Who will still ask to be seen in a park or at a dance with one who is so burned? Will a young child know this face as that of its parent, or will there be frightened wails and pleas to remove the scary mask? Who will want to touch and stroke this rough and wooden skin? Where will one know to place a kiss?

If the eyes mirror the soul, is Appel suggesting that this soul will move beyond reach? Must the spirit of one so burned turn inward after so many rebuffs and such little recognition? The face in this picture disturbs because it shows the havoc that flames on the skin can make in a life. Without its eyes this face looks directly at one who would look back, approaching the viewer in a manner that would scarcely happen on the street, in a way that screams "Look at me!" This painting affords a close-up view that tells powerfully of what such a burned face means. Never could I look upon the face of any burned patient with the intensity that I have brought to my engagement with this painting. Because the etiquette of the day-to-day forbids my steady gaze, I too will glance only lightly at one so disfigured and thus compromise my regard. But as real and disturbing as it feels to me at this moment, this burned face is art. I can look without causing embarrassment, without the risk of seeming cold or appalled.

During the time that I have spent looking, I have felt a horror of this ugliness. I have also taken into myself forever a remembrance of the pain of this soul who looks to me so that I might return the gaze. I have looked at this face through my own self-awareness, asking how this burning would affect me. I have gazed at this face as if it were mine. But in the act of imagining what this experience might be like for me, I have moved outside myself to a profound understanding of someone else. I have engaged in empathy. I have entered into another because I have engaged with this painting. I am reminded of what I first saw in this painting—flowers among thorns in a windswept desert—and I know that the next time I meet someone with a burned face I will remember this encounter with Appel's work. I will remember to look into the face, so that there will be two of us on this windswept desert.

Index

DATE DUE